If we have moved up ahead out of darkness, it is because a few have dared to walk ahead in the sun hand in hand.

Robert F. Allen's revision of a quote attributed to George Sand

Some seeds fell by the wayside, and the fowls devoured them up; some fell upon stony places... and because they had no root, they withered away. And some fell among thorns and the thorns sprung up, and choked them; but others fell into good ground, and brought forth fruit...

Matthew 13:4-8

Wellness Leadership

Creating supportive environments for healthier and more productive employees

By

Judd Allen, Ph.D.

Copyright 2008

Human Resources Institute, LLC

151 Dunder Road

Burlington, Vermont 05401

www.healthyculture.com

(802) 862-8855

Wellness Leadership: Creating Supportive Work Environments for Healthier and More Productive Employees

ISBN 978-0-94-1703-23-9

Library of Congress Control Number 2008930597

Published by

healthyculture.com

Contact information:

Human Resources Institute, LLC

151 Dunder Road

Burlington, VT 05401 USA

(802) 862-8855

Info@healthyculture.com

www.Healthyculture.com

Quantity purchases of *Wellness Leadership* are available for educational, business and community use.

Cartoon drawings by Isabella Bannerman. Ms. Bannerman also works on a newspaper comic strip, syndicated by King Features, called "Six Chix." More information is available at Isabellabannerman.com.

Cover photograph of Judd Allen by Karen Pike of www.kpikephoto.com.

Cover photograph available through Getty Images. The people shown are models used for illustrative purposes only.

Contents

Acknowledgments

Ken Holtyn, of Holtyn Associates, Inc., played a key role in researching the formation of wellness committees and the legal issues associated with worksite wellness. He has been engaged in promoting wellness for more than 20 years, and his practical experience and wisdom contributed substantially to this book.

In 1998, David Hunnicutt of Wellness Councils of America (WELCOA) offered me access to WELCOA's board of directors. Interviews with these senior executives solidified the leadership development framework incorporated into this book. The taped interviews were woven into the *Wellness Leadership* video. In 1999, Dr. Hunnicutt and I coauthored an article titled "Wellness Leadership." Building on this experience, I developed a leadership training and assessment. Subsequent interest in these resources made it possible for me to engage more than 100 organizations on this topic. Most of the content of this book was a result of the initial WELCOA Wellness Leadership project.

Garry Lindsay of Partnership for Prevention has been working with senior executives to communicate the wellness vision. Although this book is not directed specifically to executives, many of the testimonials developed by Partnership for Prevention have raised my awareness about the role leaders play in promoting wellness.

I would like to thank my friends, family, colleagues and clients for their input and enthusiasm during the writing process. I particularly thank my colleagues Troy Adams, Steve Aldana, Carol Ardell, Don Ardell, Bill Baun, Marybeth Baun, Craig Becker, James Carman, Larry Chapman, Dee Edington, Bruce Fetzer, Dennis Elsenrath, David Gobble, Bill Hettler, Joseph Leutzinger, Japie Lubbe, Michael O'Donnell, Gillian Pieper, Kay Ryan and Elaine Sullivan. These wellness experts have been especially helpful in making sure that *Wellness Leadership* is both practical and based in good science.

Thanks also to the *American Journal of Health Promotion*, Institute for Health and Productivity Management, National Wellness Institute, Partnership for Prevention, University of Michigan Health Management Research Center, Wellness Africa, WELCOA and the many businesses, communities and organizations that have embraced and tested the wellness leadership concepts.

About the Author

Judd Allen earned his Ph.D. in community psychology from New York University. He is president of the Human Resources Institute, LLC (also known as Healthyculture.com), a research, publishing and consulting firm that focuses on the creation of supportive cultural environments. He has assisted several hundred business, educational, community and government organizations in creating healthier and more productive cultures. Dr. Allen serves on the editorial board of the *American Journal of Health Promotion* and is on the board of directors of the National Wellness Institute. He has taught on the faculties of Nebraska Methodist College, Cornell University Medical College, Johnson State College and the Institute for Health and Productivity Management. Dr. Allen was a senior research analyst at Memorial Sloan-Kettering Cancer Center and has served on the Vermont Governor's Council for Physical Fitness and Sports.

He loves to travel, exercise and play with friends and family. Dr. Allen has completed more than 25 consecutive New York City Marathons as well as Ironman distance triathlons and long-distance cross-country ski races. He lives in Burlington, Vermont, with his wife and daughter.

Author Update 2010. Two organizations, Wellness Leadership Coaching and Wellness Culture Coaching, have been formed to advance wellness leadership.. Wellness Leadership Coaching provides coaching services to managers. Wellness Culture Coaching empowers wellness professionals to add culture change resources to their practices. The new companies offer wellness leadership training and coaching, as well as an exciting new management feedback system called the Wellness Leadership Dashboard. Further information is available at:

www.healthyculture.com

Chapter 1: A Call to Wellness Leadership

Our society faces an epidemic that is caused largely by unhealthy lifestyle practices. Unhealthy lifestyles are factors in the six leading causes of death – heart disease, cancer, stroke, respiratory diseases, accidents and diabetes. Together they account for 70 percent of all deaths in the United States. The cost of this epidemic in lost lives and needless suffering are widespread. The economic costs are a tremendous burden to individuals, businesses and communities.

Contrast that grim picture with the likely benefits of shifting toward wellness. Healthy lifestyles that include such elements as getting physical activity, practicing good nutrition and making time for social engagement save lives and lower costs. Healthier lifestyles also deliver vitality, the ability to focus and the capacity to achieve our full potential. Productivity and morale gains make a "well workplace" culture a primary business objective.

Wellness Leadership was written to help you effectively and efficiently support wellness among work groups. You will be creating a well workplace culture. The goal is to establish strong norms for healthy lifestyle practices and for successful lifestyle improvement. The leadership skills and practices recommended in this book will leverage your influence and increase the likelihood that members of your group will successfully achieve their wellness lifestyle goals.

Wellness Leadership is intended for anyone seeking to play a positive role in supporting wellness, including managers at all levels and wellness committee members. This book is applicable to any organization: public or private, large or small, local or widespread. Although this book is intended primarily for those engaged in work, the same leadership principles are well suited for creating supportive family and community environments.

Our Culture of Self-Improvement

Each year most of your coworkers will attempt to adopt new healthy lifestyle practices. Common goals include losing weight, managing stress, becoming physically active, stopping smoking, adopting a more positive outlook, maintaining closer friendships and controlling alcohol and other substance abuse. Motives include looking good, feeling great, becoming more productive, recovering from illness and addressing safety or health concerns. Some goals will be inspired by a news report, feedback from a health questionnaire or a conversation with a health practitioner. Encouragement from concerned friends and family members can also spark lifestyle change efforts. Many people's goals will have been on their "to do" list for some time. Some of these goals become New Year's resolutions. Other goals, set in response to a medical emergency, rapidly become an urgent priority.

Almost all employees would benefit from successful lifestyle change. The percentage of Americans who adhere to all four of the most basic lifestyle prescriptions for good health – not smoking, maintaining a healthy weight, eating adequate fruits and vegetables, and getting physical activity – is a dismal 3 percent. About two-thirds of American adults are overweight or obese. More than half (55 percent) do not get enough regular physical activity. Only 25 percent eat recommended amounts of fruits and vegetables. Substance abuse, smoking, social isolation and lack of sleep also undermine the health and well-being of many Americans.

The Wellness Challenge

Unfortunately, most lifestyle change attempts do not result in long-term behavior change. The effort is usually abandoned in the first week or month. And among those people who do make a change, few change to the extent intended. It is not uncommon for a person to try to make the same behavior change many times without success. This is called "yo-yo dieting" when it involves weight management. The same yo-yo experience is common for stopping smoking, managing stress and other lifestyle change goals. The vast majority of smokers, for example, have tried to quit multiple times. Most overweight employees have lost the same pounds repeatedly. Your unfit employees are likely to have exercise shoes and fitness equipment in their closets.

See for Yourself

Next time you are in a group of 10 or more people, ask for a show of hands…

Raise your hand if in the past year, you attempted to change one or more health practices. This includes attempts to lose weight, exercise more, manage stress, improve friendships or anything else you might have done for a New Year's resolution or other reason.

You are very likely to see a vast majority of hands go up.

Then, privately, so as not to cause embarrassment, ask about success. How many people fully achieved their lifestyle change goals? Listen to their experiences. You are very likely to hear about big plans and little progress. Most people will report that they did not fully achieve their intended goals for more than a brief time.

The wellness challenge is further compounded by the fact that the vast majority of employees have two or more unhealthy practices that need attention. Such lifestyle change will only get them off the endangered list. It is likely that they will want to add positive lifestyle goals on a regular basis to achieve optimal well-being.

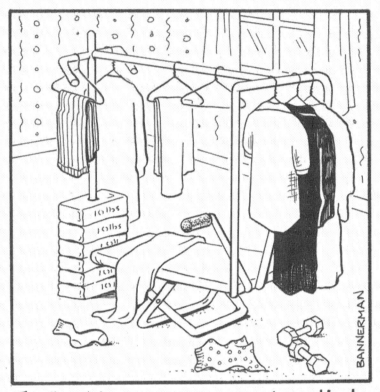

Finally. A home exercise system that really is a clothes rack!

We try to laugh off failed health resolutions and the sad state of our overall wellness, but the mental and physical health consequences are serious. Failure is stressful and undermines self-esteem. Failure also undermines our enthusiasm for wellness goals and wellness activities. As a result, many managers and physicians are reluctant to promote wellness because they do not want to set people up to fail.

To cope with our inability to change, we avoid health messages that make us feel bad about how we behave. Another common strategy is denial. We pretend that our unhealthy practices are not too bad or we deny that they make a difference to our health and well-being. Denial and inaction help us avoid public embarrassment and the added stress of lifestyle change failure.

The Demand for Workplace Wellness Programs

Wellness programs have become a financial necessity for organizations struggling to manage healthcare costs. As remarkable as it may seem, despite a high lifestyle change failure rate, wellness programs are able to earn their keep by reducing medical costs, absenteeism and turnover. Average return on investment across most industries exceeds $3 for every $1 invested. Perhaps this is not so remarkable considering what a single heart attack costs (many thousands of dollars for ambulance, diagnostics, treatment and short-term hospitalization). The savings from two fewer heart attacks more than covers the cost of a great deal of wellness programming.

The current approach to promoting wellness emphasizes initial motivation and health information. A typical offering includes a personal health survey, counseling and a health newsletter or information Web site. Annual events such as health fairs and contests are sometimes thrown into the mix. They have a "feel-good" quality that fits with a culture preoccupied with self-determination. Such efforts rarely address the underlying conditions that lead people toward unhealthy practices. Physical and social environments that work against wellness goals are typically ignored.

A Total Quality Management Perspective

Most wellness programs would not pass total quality management tests for sustained results. Employees in these programs are rarely able to maintain desired lifestyle changes. Programs with such high failure rates are unable to inspire ongoing participation or commitment of resources. Most wellness activities are done on a shoestring budget. Typical wellness program budgets are far smaller than other human resource investments, representing a tiny fraction (less than 5 percent) of expenditures on health insurance.

Many managers are aware that wellness programs lack the necessary oomph. A study of senior and middle managers in 24 companies found general agreement that adults will change a health behavior if they are supported in doing so by people they spend time with, and that changes are more likely when supportive policies are in place. Only 34 percent of these managers thought that information alone would be enough to promote healthy changes. Managers with prior wellness program experience were less likely than managers with no past program experience to believe that offering such programs would improve employee relations, or that employees would change health behavior. Based on this feedback, it appears that many managers recognize that wellness program goals are laudable. However, managers also recognize that such programs are defective in that they are unable to deliver needed change.

If a company were to increase lifestyle change success rates (from 20 percent to more than 50 percent), the wellness program would become a sought-after employee benefit and a competitive advantage. Imagine the greater savings on medical costs, lowered absenteeism and increased productivity that could be achieved by higher success rates. Higher success rates would also make the wellness program a morale builder and a source of corporate pride.

Dramatic action seems warranted. However, the obvious quick fixes are probably of little practical benefit.

- Your organization could hire people without health risks. This would narrow the applicant pool to less than 10 percent of the population.

- Your organization could fire employees with health risks. This would probably place your company in legal jeopardy. Some of these health risks are now governed by laws pertaining to business discrimination and disability. This approach would also enrage many people.

- Your organization could upgrade the quality and quantity of its motivational health information. For example, your wellness program could tailor health information to employee needs and learning styles. It could offer counselors to talk through goals with employees. Such improvements probably couldn't hurt, but it is apparent that employees are already sufficiently motivated to attempt healthy lifestyle change. Employees are already familiar with the health consequences of inaction, and many are very knowledgeable about possible change strategies.

- Your organization could pay employees to adopt healthier practices. There is little doubt that money will capture people's attention. However, people don't normally expect to be paid for brushing their teeth, eating vegetables and other personal health practices. This approach adds new meaning to the concept of working all the time. In addition, it seems unlikely that most employees can achieve lasting health behavior changes, regardless of the incentives.

- Your organization could declare that the success rate of current behavior change goals does not count and only program participation matters. Participation rates are already widely adopted standards for many wellness programs. So, for example, the program would be considered successful if a high percentage of employees completed annual health questionnaires. Lowering the bar by discounting the importance of successful lifestyle change could improve the program numbers. However, such a strategy is not directly linked to improved health and productivity. Lasting health behavior change is the most direct outcome measure.

In short, these quick fixes are not acceptable options, particularly for an initiative that is supposed to promote self-responsibility and well-being. Just as with any good quality improvement program, it is important to look at the processes and conditions that cause failure.

Stepping Up to a Well Workplace Culture Solution

Fortunately, culture change is a substantial and largely untapped mechanism for improving lifestyle change success rates and lowering risk. You can co-create a work environment that lowers physical and social barriers to healthy lifestyle choices. You can co-create a workplace culture in which it is unlikely that employees will encounter or adopt additional unhealthy practices. In a health-supporting environment, wellness activities become a part of the daily routine.

The word culture originated from the farming concept of cultivation. True to this origin, group and organizational cultures cultivate and nurture attitudes and behavior. Culture is made up of the visible and invisible social forces that shape behavior and beliefs. Families, friends, households, workplaces and communities all have cultures and subcultures. These cultures vary in terms of the beliefs and behaviors they support. The strength and rigidity of cultural influences also varies. A culture may be silent about a health behavior. A culture may also be highly proscriptive, exerting severe consequences for individual deviation from the norms. Such is the case with drug laws and work rules prohibiting the use of recreational drugs.

Cultures are complex systems of visible and less obvious social influences. Many cultural influences are subtle, operating beyond our conscious awareness. Furthermore, people get so accustomed to their cultural environments that they tend to lose track of the impact of those environments. This is called "being acculturated." Cultures adapt to the natural environment and play a large role in determining the built environment, which includes transportation, recreational facilities, workplaces and living arrangements. The culture makes cigarettes, junk food and televisions possible Cultures also make walking paths, green building construction, health foods and ergonomic workstations possible. Cultural forces interpret organizational policies and procedures and heavily influence whether they work as intended. So, for example, the written policy may be to have an hour long lunch break, but the cultural norm could be to work through lunch.

The Role of Leadership in Wellness

Organizational leaders can play an important role in fostering a well workplace culture that supports the health and well-being of employees. Executives, managers, wellness professionals and wellness committees can join together to promote a well workplace culture. *Wellness Leadership* is about making it easier for members of your work group to practice healthy lifestyles of their own choosing. It is about removing barriers to success. It is not about telling others how to behave, but rather describes how to create conditions that support people in their quest for health and happiness.

Management efforts to nurture a supportive environment fall into four broad and overlapping leadership responsibilities. *Wellness Leadership* addresses knowledge and skills related to:

- **Sharing the Wellness Vision.** Your explanation for why wellness is important, how people can get personally involved and what the organization is doing to make it easier for people to achieve healthier lifestyles.

- **Serving as Role Models.** Your capacity to visibly demonstrate a commitment to wellness through your own behavior and participation. Your actions speak volumes and will inspire others.

- **Aligning Cultural Touch Points.** Your efforts to adjust organizational policies and procedures to support wellness. Influences such as the physical environment, rewards, feedback and training play important roles in supporting wellness behavior. Such adjustments also help eliminate barriers to positive practices.

- **Monitoring and Celebrating Success.** Your efforts to track wellness so that collective and individual progress can be recognized. Your attention and encouragement make it easier to stay on track with lasting and positive behavior change.

Wellness Leadership offers a framework for thinking about and organizing your support for wellness. Four chapters explore leadership skills. A fifth chapter discusses the special roles of executives, wellness professionals and wellness committees in organizing the wellness program. Pick those subjects that are of greatest interest or read the book through to develop a complete skill set. These leadership skills, when combined with your practical know-how, creativity, inspiration and persistence, are likely to play a powerful and positive role in creating a well workplace culture.

Most managers are already working to support the well-being of their employees. This book builds on your current efforts to promote employee well-being by taking a closer look at several powerful environmental support strategies. *Wellness Leadership* shows you how to refine these efforts. See how you are doing in supporting a well workplace culture by filling out The Wellness Leadership Indicator.

The Wellness Leadership Indicator

Rate your level of agreement with the following statements on the 5-point scale: (5) strongly agree, (4) agree, (3) undecided/don't know, (2) disagree, and (1) strongly disagree.

I consistently:

5 4 3 2 1	Describe the wellness program in a way that employees understand.
5 4 3 2 1	Express enthusiasm for the wellness initiative.
5 4 3 2 1	Share how I personally benefit from wellness.
5 4 3 2 1	Help employees see how they may personally benefit from wellness.
5 4 3 2 1	Discuss why wellness is among the top organizational priorities.
5 4 3 2 1	Explain how employees can participate in the wellness effort.
5 4 3 2 1	Ask for employee input about the wellness effort.
5 4 3 2 1	Make lifestyle choices that demonstrate my commitment to wellness.
5 4 3 2 1	Participate in the wellness program.
5 4 3 2 1	Eliminate or reduce barriers to healthy lifestyles.
5 4 3 2 1	Recruit employees who are open to pursuing wellness.
5 4 3 2 1	See to it that new people are aware of the wellness program.

The Wellness Leadership Indicator Continued

Rate your level of agreement with the following statements on the 5-point scale: (5) strongly agree, (4) agree, (3) undecided/don't know, (2) disagree, and (1) strongly disagree.

I consistently:

5 4 3 2 1	See to it that people are taught skills needed to achieve their wellness goals.
5 4 3 2 1	Establish wellness traditions and rituals.
5 4 3 2 1	See to it that individuals get regular lifestyle assessments.
5 4 3 2 1	See to it that work teams are given collective feedback regarding wellness.
5 4 3 2 1	Use wellness activities for team building.
5 4 3 2 1	See to it that adequate time, space, and other resources are available for wellness practices.
5 4 3 2 1	Reward and recognize individuals for their wellness efforts.
5 4 3 2 1	Reward and recognize groups and work teams for their collective wellness efforts.

How did you do? There are 20 questions and a possible total score of 100. Don't be discouraged if your answers reflect only modest support for employees' wellness. These questions are likely to be different from what you are accustomed to in that they examine your efforts to create conditions for pursuing wellness. *Wellness Leadership* was written to build on your leadership strengths and your capacity to positively influence others.

Leadership Stories

◆ Aphra's work group has been under a lot of pressure. She's seen her team shrink in size, but the demands have increased. Technology and innovation have raised individual productivity, but everyone must be on their toes in order to keep up. The last thing Aphra wants is to add to employees' "to do" lists. Wellness looks like a good idea, but only if integrated seamlessly into the hectic work schedule.

◆ Ray is embarrassed about his weight. He's a veteran of many failed diets. He completed the health assessment at work, and the feedback was nothing new. As he told his coworkers, "If they really cared, they would change the cafeteria and vending-machine selections." That just got the complaints rolling. It seemed obvious to everyone that the company's wellness program lacked any real follow-through.

◆ Eileen knows that more will need to be done to promote wellness. Eileen has served on her company's wellness committee since the wellness program began in 1980. She has seen many good ideas come and go. In the early days, the program featured support groups and wellness classes. After a decade, stress management workshops, smoking cessation classes and parenting support groups gave way to an emphasis on health information. A wellness newsletter and then a Web site offered the latest lifestyle recommendations. A few years ago, the program was revamped again so that activities are linked back to personal health assessments. Those with more lifestyle risks get telephone coaching. However, it has become increasingly difficult to get employees to participate. The company now offers a discount on health insurance co-payments in exchange for completing the health assessment. As one employee put it, "Now they're bribing us." Eileen wonders about the prospects for the latest strategy.

◆Tyler markets his hospital's wellness services to area businesses. His clients are willing to commit only to basic activities such as the health newsletter and an occasional seminar. Apparently, they have fairly low expectations about what a wellness program can achieve. He knows that his clients are alarmed by escalating health insurance and disability costs. Tyler would like to find a way to reengage the decision makers, but so far they seem uninterested.

Chapter 2: Creating a Shared Wellness Vision

Characteristics of a Shared Vision

Have you been in a group or organization with a strong shared vision? The classic example occurred at NASA when President Kennedy set a goal of putting a man on the moon. Another example took place during the civil rights era when Martin Luther King talked about his dream of eliminating racial discrimination. In both instances, people pulled together to accomplish substantial goals. These goals were so grand that they required a level of faith, hope and hard work that would have been unimaginable without visionary leadership. Fortunately, a shared vision of this magnitude and scope is not normally required for a successful worksite wellness initiative. However, an inspired shared vision will go a long way toward success.

A distinctive feature of a shared vision is that it touches people on a personal level. The following experiences are common to shared visions. A shared vision exists when:

- **People are inspired by the purpose of the effort.** A shared vision is said to be inspirational when it is seen as worthy of considerable effort. People have genuine enthusiasm for what is being accomplished. The goals, direction, and approach stimulate excitement that goes beyond ordinary tasks.

- **People feel that their values and ideas are incorporated into what the organization is trying to achieve.** People need to see how their personal values and priorities are taken into consideration. People recognize how input was collected and incorporated into the effort. It is not so much that the vision has to match individual priorities exactly. Rather, it is important that personal input was taken into consideration.

- **People can easily communicate the mission and direction of the effort.** The vision must be summarized in such a way that people can explain what it's all about. This does not mean that the vision is easy or uncomplicated, but rather that it is explained in a highly understandable and accessible way. People with a shared vision need to see the big picture as well as how it looks from their vantage point.

- **People recognize that both individual and organizational needs are being addressed.** For example, a workplace wellness program offers cost savings and enhanced human performance. In a similar way, those carrying the vision forward must see personal benefits. Benefits could occur in the form of better health, greater personal safety or increased feelings of wellness. The result is a win-win whereby the success of the individual enhances the likely benefits to the group. Similarly, the success of the group has obvious and direct payoffs to individuals.

- **People see how their day-to-day activities can support the overall goals of the effort.** Shared visions are participatory. This is something we do together. People must be able to see their roles and their contribution to success.

Notice that a shared vision differs substantially from normal business practices and objectives. Most organizations and employees have a "to do" list of tasks to be accomplished in the course of regular business. For example, employees need to be hired and trained. Customer orders need to be placed and invoiced. Products must be built and delivered. A shared vision differs in that it sets forth a special purpose that calls for a higher level of attention, inventiveness, teamwork and commitment.

A well workplace requires a shared vision because wellness philosophies and lifestyles are substantial departures from common practice. A well workplace is not achieved simply through wellness activities such as completing health assessments, reading health newsletters and speaking to wellness coaches. A wellness program could include any or all of these activities, but a shared vision for a well workplace goes beyond a menu of wellness activities. A well workplace is a way of doing business that puts optimal employee health and well-being on the high-priority list alongside such goals as profitability, outstanding customer service and new product innovation. A well workplace positively influences employee wellness by adjusting business practices in such a way that employee health and well-being are integral to how work gets done.

Successful wellness programs create a vibrant, inspiring and useful vision of the wellness initiative. The wellness vision must be tailored to fit the organization's language, needs and traditions. It must inspire your work teams and individual employees. Your goal is to paint a clear picture of wellness in the workplace that inspires employees to seek wellness in their own lives and to make good use of wellness opportunities at the worksite. Your enthusiastic explanation of the wellness initiative must be heartfelt.

Establishing Wellness Roots in Your Workplace Culture

Wellness is a relatively new concept that can easily be misunderstood. There are, for example, many products and services that now include "wellness" in their name or description. Unless you want your efforts to be confused with a new spa treatment, a chiropractic visit or some other holistic practice, you will need to clarify what wellness means in your organization.

A Brief History of the Wellness Philosophy

The National Wellness Institute (NWI) defines wellness as a conscious, self-directed and evolving process of achieving full potential (see www.nationalwellness.org). The NWI definition also states that wellness is multidimensional and holistic, encompassing lifestyle, mental and spiritual well-being and the environment. According to NWI, wellness is positive and affirming. This definition has remained relatively constant over the past 25-plus years. This life philosophy has been contrasted with other approaches to health that emphasize survival and treating disease as opposed to thriving, attaining overall well-being and achieving potential. Another hallmark of the wellness philosophy has been its perspective that humans are more than the sum of their parts. Mind, body and spirit interact in such a way that it is necessary to see and address all. Wellness is seen as a positive and affirming philosophy in that it addresses potentials, process and empowerment. Within this philosophy, an individual human being and group are works in progress that always have room for growth. The wellness philosophy holds that individuals and groups are responsible for being proactive in seizing opportunities to nurture and achieve their potential.

The wellness philosophy was first articulated in the 1950s when Dr. Halbert L. Dunn, a retired public health service physician, began lecturing about what he called "high level wellness." A series of 29 lectures on this topic delivered at the Washington, D.C.,

Unitarian Church were printed in 1961. Dr. Dunn stressed the importance of mind/body/spirit connections, the need for personal satisfactions and valued purposes, and a view of health as dramatically more than non-illness. Dr. John Travis was influenced by Dr. Dunn's work when, in the 1970s, he created the Wellness Resource Center, the first clinic that focused on personal wellness. During the 1970s, Dr. Travis wrote the *Wellness Workbook*, which offered a multidimensional model of well-being. Dr. Don Ardell later popularized the wellness concept in his 1977 book, *High Level Wellness: An Alternative to Doctors, Drugs and Disease*. Also in 1977, my father, Dr. Robert Allen, wrote *Lifegain*, which examined the role of cultural support for wellness lifestyles and explained how wellness programs could be developed for households, workplaces and communities. Dr. William Hettler was the first to develop a wellness program for an academic setting, the University of Wisconsin, Stevens Point. This campus was the site of the first National Wellness Conference in 1976. Stevens Point continues to host the annual July conference as well as the National Wellness Institute.

Discovering Your Organization's Wellness History

Your organization may have a history that relates to wellness. You can use this history to explain wellness. The following questions are useful in revealing the story of wellness in your organization.

- What were the people and purposes that brought your group or organization together? Did your founder(s) have a wellness philosophy? Was mutual support or a struggle for well-being a part of this early story? Did your early days as an organization relate in some way to wellness?

- Were there some rough patches and important challenges that your company or work group had to overcome? Did this story involve courageous acts, cooperation, creativity and perseverance? These are wellness traits.

- Many products have a health and wellness aspect. Do your products or services make the world a better place, enhance health or make life more enjoyable?

- What activities, symbols and traditions make your group or organization special? Do any of these have a health or wellness aspect?

- Wellness concerns how we help others achieve their potential. Were there times your group was particularly thoughtful or caring? This could be a wellness story.

- Almost all organizations depend on the efforts and abilities of their people. This is a wellness story. How have your people made you successful?

An Example of One Company's Wellness Story

Johnson & Johnson (J&J) is a good example of a company with deep wellness roots. More than 60 years ago, the founders of J&J adopted a credo that was all about caring for the health and well-being of customers, employees, shareholders and the broader community. The J&J Credo drives the company wellness program as the program has become an extension of how to serve J&J stakeholders.

Hopefully, wellness has deep roots in your organization. Many organizations have wellness programs that date back as far as the 1970s. Even if your wellness program is new, your organization is likely to have a long history of helping its employees address quality-of-life and health issues. Your description of the wellness program should reference how a philosophy of health and human potential evolved in your organization. It is also helpful to frame your current vision as a part of national and global efforts to advance the wellness concept.

> **Learning Assignment**
>
> **Discover Your Organization's Wellness Story**
>
> Investigate past efforts that have focused on employee well-being and performance. How has a philosophy of health and human potential evolved in your organization?
>
> Record your organization's wellness story. This history will help show that the current initiative has roots.

Sharing the Wellness Value Proposition

Wellness offers many benefits to individuals and groups in addition to cost savings. Some of these benefits relate to individual health and others address organizational needs. They are a direct result of lifestyle choices and positive attitudes. The following list illustrates many of the reasons individuals and organizations are attracted to the wellness philosophy and develop activities that support wellness.

- **Reduce Health Risks.** Those people who eliminate unhealthy practices such as smoking and adopt positive practices such as physical activity are at lower risk for getting sick.

- **Control Illness Care/Costs.** Some medical costs are best reduced by lowering the demand for illness care. Healthy lifestyles reduce the likelihood of needing such care. In addition, some of the least expensive remedies involve changing behaviors, for example, stopping smoking, becoming more physically active, sleeping more or eating a healthier diet.

- **Heal.** Most chronic conditions, injuries and illnesses respond better to treatment when the medicine is combined with healthier lifestyle practices. Attitudes and behavior have important roles in the healing process.

- **Deliver Peak Performance.** Top athletes and outstanding workers continue to deliver when their minds and bodies are fit. In contrast, a lack of wellness can drag down even the most gifted. You can't work as well when you are not feeling well.

- **Achieve Full Potential/Wholeness.** Feeling great goes well beyond basic survival. Each person can achieve a higher total quality of life that optimizes his or her abilities.

- **Provide Opportunities to Assist.** Wellness affords many opportunities to help others achieve positive goals. Such kindness provides health and self-esteem benefits for the person offering assistance and the recipient of that assistance.

- **Enhance Teamwork/Morale.** Achieving healthy lifestyles cuts across common organizational barriers. Prejudices and racism can be undercut when people are brought together to work on wellness. Wellness provides opportunities for mutual support and common experience. Wellness can be uplifting even when other environmental and economic conditions are less than delightful.

- **Look Good/Improve Image.** Some people will find the ability to make themselves look healthier and more fit very appealing. In addition, organizations that support wellness demonstrate their commitment to the well-being of their employees and show good corporate citizenship. Perhaps your organization would like to enhance its public image or its appeal to customers.

Fortunately, it is not necessary to pick and choose among these benefits. The very same health behaviors that lead to a longer life expectancy appear to make it easier for people to be more productive. Some combination of the wellness value propositions is likely to resonate with almost all members of the workforce. People driven by the bottom line will be most interested in the medical cost savings and increased productivity. Others will find improving their quality of life, looking good and reaching peak performance appealing. Still others will be drawn to the social opportunities and stronger teamwork. Help your people to see the many benefits. This is not an either/or situation whereby enthusiasm for one set of benefits somehow diminishes the value of the other benefits. For example, an executive may be delighted about saving lives, enhancing teamwork and saving money. Tailor your wellness message to highlight those benefits that are most appealing to your audience.

Learning Assignment

Explore and Explain the Wellness Value Proposition

Review the list of wellness benefits.

What will you do to increase awareness of the benefits of wellness?

Making the Business Case

American business culture has a history of emphasizing capital expenditures (e.g., buildings and equipment) over human resources investment (e.g., training, health insurance and wellness programs). As a result, limited funding is available for human resource priorities. Wellness initiatives must go head-to-head with well-established human resources priorities such as job training and health insurance. Wellness leaders must be able to explain why scarce financial resources should be allocated to support wellness.

The economic benefits of wellness are achieved in a variety of ways. A successful wellness program is likely to result in:

- **Lowered absenteeism.** It is estimated that just over half of illnesses are the result of lifestyle. For example, smokers are more likely to get colds, and overweight people are more likely to have back and knee problems.

- **Reduced medical costs.** A side benefit of fewer illnesses is the ability to reduce the need for medical care. With medical costs skyrocketing, the best way to save is to lower the demand.

- **Improved productivity.** It is hard to work when you have a headache, back pain or some other ailment. Healthy lifestyle practices prevent such distracting aches and pains. Positive practices such as exercise also enhance alertness and other forms of work readiness.

- **Lower turnover.** Replacing sick and dying employees is costly. Training replacement workers can be very expensive. Employees' premature retirement can also adversely impact customer relationships.

- **Fewer accidents.** Unhealthy lifestyle practices such as substance abuse and lack of sleep increase the likelihood of accidents. Wellness can cut the risks.

- **Enhanced public image.** Many businesses earn and sell more if they are seen as responsible corporate citizens that are sensitive to public health. This is particularly true of healthcare providers, insurers and those that make health products. Public image is also a factor in any business involved in travel, consumer products or food. Nonprofit and for-profit companies depend on a healthy image to secure favorable shareholder, donor and customer preferences.

Each health practice has financial implications for your organization. One University of Michigan study of 7,026 employees found that each health risk identified in a health risk appraisal was commensurate with a 1.9 percent loss in productivity. This study valued each risk as costing $950 per year.

The importance of investing in wellness also becomes apparent through return on investment (ROI) calculations. A recent review of wellness program ROI studies found an average of more than $3 return for every $1 invested. Few other human resources initiatives have such a positive financial track record. Although the unique circumstances of your organization may differ from the many businesses that have already been studied, it is highly likely that your wellness program is a reasonable investment.

The economic evidence for wellness is strong, but don't be lulled into a false belief that promoting wellness has a guaranteed return. Visible benefits materialize only if employees are successful in achieving healthy lifestyles. To get a meaningful level of change, you must invest in wellness by creating a supportive environment. This includes aligning many of the policies and procedures of your organization to better support healthy lifestyles. Without the follow-through available in a supportive environment, few people will achieve wellness goals, and most of the benefits will not materialize. Furthermore, a wellness program makes sense only if the organization is going to make a substantial investment. A good ROI becomes powerful if the investment is there. For a $1 investment, $3.50 back is hardly worth noting. But a $400-per-employee annual expenditure is notable when it returns $1,400 per employee (a 3.5-to-1 ROI).

You must develop your own metrics for assessing the financial impact of wellness, but don't get carried away. Be careful not to require that wellness programs offer advanced proof for an economic return on investment. Few business investments are sure bets, and no other human resources initiative is held to a rigid standard of proof. Unfortunately, the research budget for some wellness programs exceeds that spent on actually helping people pursue their wellness goals. Fortunately, there is good evidence that wellness is a sound investment. There are regular reviews of this evidence in the *American Journal of Health Promotion* and at the Art and Science of Health Promotion Conference sponsored by the journal (see www. healthpromotionjournal.com). Use this evidence to build your business case.

Learning Assignment
Explore and Explain the Business Case

Review available information about the financial costs of unhealthy lifestyles.

How would healthier employees improve the bottom line?

What are your strongest arguments that economic benefits will be realized?

Shifting Attitudes toward Wellness

Members of your group will have attitudes toward wellness that range from wildly enthusiastic to totally skeptical. The following diagram illustrates this range of opinions.

Attitudes toward Wellness

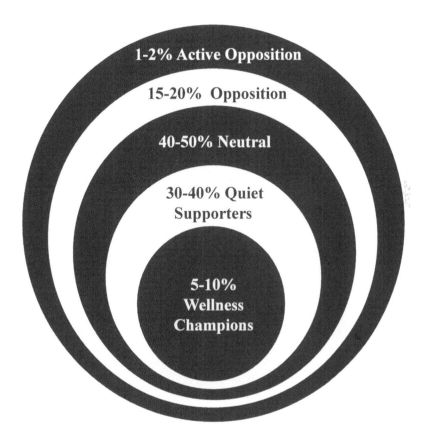

1-2% Active Opposition

15-20% Opposition

40-50% Neutral

30-40% Quiet Supporters

5-10% Wellness Champions

Slightly different approaches are needed to address the various attitudes toward wellness. The wellness champion group consists of people who, like you, think wellness is worth having. These people need your encouragement and resources to be most effective. Another important group is the quiet supporters. They are excited about wellness and have yet to find a way to contribute. Your best approach with these people is to help them see how they can make a difference through their own personal conduct and by assisting with the wellness initiative. Those who are neutral may have other concerns on their minds. This group should be encouraged to gain a clearer understanding of wellness and the many benefits wellness has to offer. With a little creativity, this group's concerns can be addressed through a wellness initiative. So, for example, a person interested in financial security may find the cost savings available through wellness appealing.

It is important not to antagonize people who are opposed to wellness. Address their concerns and assure these people that they will not be inconvenienced by the wellness effort. You could offer information that addresses some of their concerns or, at least, that balances these concerns against wellness benefits. Your goal with the active opposition is to make them less inclined to work against your wellness efforts. One strategy with this group is to acknowledge their concerns, express your conviction that they have a right to disagree and let them have their say. Do not spend a great deal of energy on this group, as your efforts may serve only to further antagonize them. Let a shift in the broader culture do the work for you. If your efforts are successful, the active opposition will become less vocal.

> ## Learning Assignment
> ## Shifting Attitudes toward Wellness
>
> Identify how members of your work group feel about wellness.
>
> What will you do to shift people toward the wellness champion position?

Addressing Concerns about Wellness

There are reasonable concerns about workplace wellness programs. Wellness leaders must acknowledge these concerns and suggest some strategies for addressing them. The following chart offers common concerns about wellness and some possible responses.

Wellness Program Concern	Possible Responses
If people wanted to live a healthy lifestyle, they would do it.	Each year most people attempt to improve their wellness and are unable to achieve their goals. Barriers and lack of support make long-term change unlikely. Our program will offer ongoing support that will break this cycle of failure.
Personal behavior is a private matter and businesses should refrain from getting involved.	Personal behavior is indeed a private matter. Privacy should be maintained while providing assistance. The focus of wellness is on making it easier for people to succeed in lifestyle goals of their own choosing.
There are laws governing wellness activities and privacy. How do leaders stay out of trouble?	Fortunately, most actions that create health-supporting environments do not require individual self-disclosure. They focus more on group activities and changes to the physical environment. Appendix B explains the laws governing this kind of activity and how you can avoid problems.
Most people do not have the time to pursue wellness.	Time is an important barrier to almost any goal. Therefore, wellness efforts focus on creating work and home environments where it is easy and convenient to practice a health lifestyle. In addition, wellness programs must be offered in a variety of time-efficient formats.

Wellness Program Concern	Possible Responses
We cannot afford wellness programs.	Fortunately, wellness programs have a reasonable and predictable cost that is well below that of other human resources benefits such as health insurance. The human and economic costs of illness are so high that wellness initiatives almost always pay for themselves.
You can't change people's behavior without changing the broader society.	Problems in the broader society do make wellness difficult for all of us. There is an epidemic of poor health practices that threatens to bankrupt the country and lower our quality of life. We can create a wellness-promoting environment at the workplace. This will help. We can simultaneously support wellness in the broader community.

Hopefully, you will see how the advantages of offering a worksite wellness program make such an effort worthwhile. The challenge is to acknowledge the downside risks and address them without draining enthusiasm for the wellness initiative.

Learning Assignment
Addressing Objections

Discuss your work group's concerns and how they might be taken into consideration.

What are the concerns about wellness in your work group, and how might they be addressed?

The Statement of Commitment

Organizational leaders are often willing to make a clear declaration that wellness is a priority. Such a statement of commitment is most likely to be heard if it comes directly from the top. Executives, union officials and other key decision makers need to find an effective way to communicate their enthusiasm and commitment for the wellness effort. Such statements can be made in written communication, at employee gatherings and on video. A statement of commitment can be incorporated into the annual report, wellness program materials and media events. You can help make sure these statements are heard.

A leadership statement is a good start. Most groups, however, have a mental litmus test for determining whether a program is more than just talk. You can learn more about this standard by asking employees to identify what the organization would need to do to show that it is really serious about wellness. In some settings, the answer would be offering fitness facilities. Alternatively, employees might say that if the company really cared, it would offer showers. In another setting, time would be the test; employees would need to be given flexible schedules for participating in wellness activities. Ideally, the organization will find a way to demonstrate commitment by passing the litmus test. If this is not possible, it will be necessary to find other ways to show commitment.

Employees need to know that the commitment to wellness will be sustained. Hiring a staff and building facilities are ways of declaring a lasting commitment. Another strategy is to develop a business-like approach to planning, implementing and evaluating the wellness initiative. Some wellness programs adopt a yearly cycle for this purpose. The program plan shows that wellness is rooted in current realities and ready to adapt to future needs. Annual rituals such as walking and running events add to the sense that wellness is an established tradition.

Learning Assignment
Broadcasting Leadership Commitment

Develop your strategy for getting your work group to appreciate that organizational leaders are fully behind the initiative.

How will you see to it that the commitment is made and heard?

What will be done to show that the program is more than just words?

How will you make it clear that the commitment is ongoing?

Wellness Dimensions and Themes

Although generally people have a positive sense that wellness is related to full potential, quality of life and health, most people have not fully formed a definition of wellness. Most people are willing to entertain new ideas as to how wellness works. Individuals and groups can define wellness in a way that is vital and relevant to changing needs. Such openness makes wellness an ideal word for creating a shared vision. People can come together to define wellness in a way that is most meaningful and helpful.

There are many valid themes for wellness. Some organizations, for example, focus on physical wellness. These organizations emphasize such themes as healthy eating, physical activity, medical self-care and the avoidance of substance abuse. Such wellness programs are often called "population health management," "health and productivity management" or "health promotion." Other organizations emphasize worksite safety within their wellness program. A program like this could include such goals as fatigue management and elimination of alcohol abuse. The proper use of safety equipment and emergency preparedness would also be subjects for worksite safety initiatives.

Many organizations adopt a wellness definition with a special emphasis that is true to tradition and needs. For example, the integrated energy company ConocoPhillips went with an emphasis on pleasure when it determined that its previous health risk management theme was not energizing the employees. Wellness was organized around increasing personal enjoyment. Ben & Jerry's Homemade Ice Cream went with a theme of fun. Company leaders felt that fun fit better with their product and image. At Ben & Jerry's, wellness became a matter of keeping life and work lively.

Learning Assignment
Determining Your Organization's Wellness Themes

Inquire about the themes of your wellness program. Possible people to ask include members of the wellness committee, a wellness professional or human resources professionals. If such themes are unavailable, invent them.

What theme(s) define your wellness initiative?

Setting Norm Goals

Cultural norms can be described as "the way we do things around here." They are sometimes written rules, but they are more likely to be unwritten. Norms about physical activity, healthy eating, stress management, safety and other health behaviors frequently go unnoticed until they are violated. For example, it is likely that anyone driving a few miles below the speed limit would receive special attention on the road. This safe practice goes against the common practice of driving at or above the speed limit and is likely to annoy other drivers.

Successful wellness programs establish or strengthen norms for healthy lifestyle choices. So, for example, it could become a strong norm for railroad workers not to drink alcohol before their night shift. Such drinking would be quickly confronted and brought to the attention of the employee assistance program.

An important wellness leadership responsibility is to set forth which health behaviors will become normal practice. You should work with members of your group and those responsible for coordinating the wellness program to agree upon such behavioral norm goals. These norm goals set forth how the culture will take a stand in support of wellness. These norms are how members of the culture will "walk the talk" when it comes to wellness. In the "Aligning Cultural Touch Points" chapter, you will learn how to establish and maintain these wellness norms.

Learning Assignment
Identifying Wellness Norm Goals

Review the priorities of the wellness program and the needs of your work group to determine which two or three health practices should be the focus.

What positive practices should become cultural norms in the first round of culture change?

What norm goals should be the focus of future rounds of culture change?

Inviting Participation

Your leadership role includes describing how to participate as well as how to get further information. This involves being able to explain how the program is evaluated (see the "Monitoring and Celebrating Success" chapter). You should also be able to describe what is being done to create a more supportive environment (see the "Aligning Cultural Touch Points" chapter). Ideally, you should help employees access updated information. Such information may be available in a wellness newsletter or at a wellness Web site.

Your employees need to understand that you see their participation as worthwhile. Try to reduce barriers to participation. This may require that you work with your employees to make sure that job responsibilities are taken into consideration. Perhaps a flexible schedule or some other arrangement can be made so that employees can participate without undermining their work.

Learning Assignment
Inviting Participation

Develop your plan for inviting participation.

How will you stay current about wellness program initiatives?

How will you keep your team informed?

What will you do to reduce barriers to participation?

Creating a Shared Wellness Vision Checklist

Before turning to the next chapter on serving as an effective role model, make sure you have built a good wellness leadership foundation. The following checklist will help you determine whether you have covered the core leadership opportunities   associated with sharing the wellness vision.

☐ **Tell your organization's wellness story.** How is the wellness initiative rooted in the history of your organization? Why will wellness contribute to a brighter future?

☐ **Tell employees about all the benefits that could result from a well workplace.** Which wellness benefits do you find most appealing and why?

Creating a Shared Wellness Vision Checklist

Before turning to the next chapter on serving as an effective role model, make sure you have built a good wellness leadership foundation. The following checklist will help you determine whether you have covered the core leadership opportunities associated with sharing the wellness vision.

☐ **Tell your organization's wellness story.** How is the wellness initiative rooted in the history of your organization? Why will wellness contribute to a brighter future?

☐ **Tell employees about all the benefits that could result from a well workplace.** Which wellness benefits do you find most appealing and why?

☐ **Discuss the business case for wellness.** What economic issues are addressed by the wellness program? How could the wellness program improve the economic outlook for employees and the organization?

☐ **Discuss how you will size up your employees' attitudes toward wellness.** How will you move people toward becoming wellness champions?

☐ **Discuss your employees' concerns about offering a workplace wellness program.** What steps can you take to address these concerns?

☐ **Discuss the commitment being made to wellness.** How will you inform your work group about this commitment? Who will have primary responsibility and oversight for the initiative? What is being done to demonstrate that this is a serious commitment? What is the long-term plan?

☐ **Offer a definition of wellness that you think best meets your organization's needs.** What are the core themes and principles of the wellness initiative? Try to keep your definition short and inspirational. This will make it easier to explain and remember.

☐ **Discuss your wellness norm goals.** What new wellness practices will become "the way we do things around here"?

☐ **Discuss how employees are to participate in the wellness program.** What are the core activities that everyone should do? What options are available to interested employees? How will your people stay informed about wellness program developments?

Leadership Stories

◆ At first it seemed like a joke. How could a convenience food company declare a commitment to wellness? However, the marketing department knew that the public was clamoring for healthy alternatives. Company owners did not want their family business to lose its "good citizen" image. New and healthier products were in the pipeline, and the employee wellness program was ready to launch. It was going to take some doing, but the company was no stranger to change.

◆ The merger was going through. At first, Dr. Andrews, the new dean, had no idea how to pull together such a diverse and widespread student body. She carefully listened for what the university and students really wanted. The students wanted jobs upon graduation. The administration and faculty wanted to lose the college's reputation as a party school. What if the school were to use wellness as a strategic advantage in selling its graduates to employers? Employers would know that each graduate was truly fit for work. The idea quickly caught fire. Faculty, administration and students embraced the vision of using the merger to create a new wellness culture.

◆ The hospital had an entire catalog devoted to wellness programs: a lot of activities, but no common thread. Johan, the director of wellness, decided it was time to regain focus. According to employee surveys and interviews, stress and work/life balance were big concerns. New norms for using work breaks were needed. Another norm was needed that would keep the work week to 40 hours. Creating cultural support for work/life balance would be the focus of this year's new wellness initiatives.

◆ Maria noticed that a yearly planning cycle worked best at her assembly plant. It gave the wellness program a rhythm and logical order. In the fall, assessments were completed. The last weeks of December were used to celebrate the year's accomplishments and to set forth next year's goals. Employees liked to use January to kick off their New Year's health resolutions. New wellness policies and procedures were also introduced early in the year. Support groups, classes and wellness coaching were in high demand during the late winter and early spring. Family activities were in full swing during the summer months.

◆ Andreas and his leadership team demanded that wellness undergo a total quality improvement transformation. Quality had become the buzzword within the entire multi-site health care organization. A recent employee survey had found that less than 20 percent of lifestyle change efforts were successful. The executive committee set this year's target success rate at 50 percent. The worksite wellness program would be reorganized for maximum support. Once an employee declared his or her goal, it would be a shared responsibility to make it work. Barriers would be reduced or eliminated. The best coaching and training would be made available. Coworkers, managers, family members and friends would all be engaged in creating the best conditions for success.

Chapter 3: Serving as an Effective Role Model

In the previous chapter, you helped develop the vision for a well workplace. The wellness definition and themes set forth a vision for a well workplace culture. You identified norm goals and health behaviors that would be the focus of the current initiative. You determined ways that employees could engage in this wellness vision. Your efforts to serve as an effective role model should build on the wellness vision. You can make choices that "walk the talk." As can be seen in the following examples, there are many ways you can serve as an effective wellness role model, and none of them require that you become a superathlete or the perfect human specimen.

- **Make Your Strengths Visible.** If you are like most people, you are already engaged in a number of positive health practices. Ideally, your current behavior overlaps with the healthy practices that are the current focus of your wellness initiative. These strengths could inspire others. At the very least, your positive practices will give others permission to try adopting similar health behavior. Many coworkers will be unaware of your wellness activities. Your employees might benefit from realizing that you have adopted these positive practices. They may also benefit from your experience with these strengths, including learning how they were developed and how these practices have played a positive role in your life.

- **Make Your Wellness Goals Visible**. Your wellness goals and your efforts to achieve these goals could be a source of inspiration for employees. This is particularly important if your current practices are not in accord with wellness program objectives. Your attitude about changing your unhealthy practices sends a clear message that it is OK to pursue wellness. Pick one or two goals that are likely to visibly demonstrate your commitment to wellness. The goals should be heartfelt and meaningful to you. They need not be the most difficult to achieve nor the most pressing. However, they should be goals that you would feel comfortable discussing with others. Being an effective role model is a public undertaking.

- **Find Ways to Participate.** With luck, your wellness goals lend themselves to participating in the wellness program. Such participation might include signing up for assessments and coaching, attending support group programs and making use of health information resources. Your participation is one of your ongoing management responsibilities. Schedule wellness participation into your weekly routine. Your attendance and participation will influence others to take advantage of wellness programming. It will also be a great morale boost to those involved in the wellness effort.

- **Don't Publicize Your Weaknesses or Your Resistance to Change.** It's OK if you have some unhealthy practices and yet are satisfied with the way things stand. Try not to press others to adopt similar unhealthy practices. You could also attempt to reduce the visibility of these behaviors by practicing them in private or out of sight. This will reduce any negative role modeling effects.

Qualities of an Effective Wellness Role Model

An effective role model provides inspiration, insight, encouragement and an appreciation of the many benefits of successful change. You can enhance your positive influence by becoming a more effective role model. The following table describes role modeling practices to develop and those to avoid.

Qualities of an Effective Role Model	Qualities of an Ineffective Role Model
Recognizes that great benefits were realized through successful lifestyle change.	Views his own change efforts as more trouble than they were worth.
Is willing to share her story, including the difficult parts.	Shares nothing about personal experience beyond that it was successful.
Sees change as a process.	Expects quick fixes.
Is not quick to criticize or to judge.	Immediately makes character judgments.
Believes it is important to get support from others and shares how other people played a role in her success.	Thinks change is best achieved without the support or involvement of others.
Acknowledges that change can be a challenge.	Says that change is easy.
Gives others permission to create their own path to success.	Recognizes only one way to success: "my way."

Conducting a Lifestyle Strength Review

When making personal changes and when serving as a role model, it is helpful to be aware of personal strengths and personal goals. The following *Wellness Lifestyle Inventory* helps to assess your current strengths, your opportunities for improvement and your interest in change. It helps determine needs and priorities. It covers a broad range of possible goals within the areas of emotional, spiritual, physical, economic and social wellness.

Wellness Lifestyle Inventory

Instructions: For each wellness practice, answer two questions. First, determine whether or not you perform the practice already. Check the boxes for these strengths. Then decide whether or not you would like to change this aspect of your life. In the column labeled "Satisfaction," check the boxes associated with areas you would like to change.

EMOTIONAL & SPIRITUAL-WELLNESS	Achievement	Satisfaction
Rate your achievement and personal satisfaction with your current wellness.	**Yes, I already do this**	**I would like to change this**
Start your day rested and with a good attitude.	☐	☐
Rarely feel "blue."	☐	☐
Achieve a balance between work, rest and play.	☐	☐
Balance work and family/household responsibilities.	☐	☐
Rarely feel stress (less than a few times a week).	☐	☐
Take time during most days for prayer, meditation or reflection.	☐	☐
Feel your life is important.	☐	☐
Use personal mistakes as opportunities to learn and grow.	☐	☐
Rarely take personal offense.	☐	☐
View most problems as temporary and manageable.	☐	☐
Be in control of your own behavior.	☐	☐
Feel that you are basically a good person.	☐	☐
Feel good about how your body looks.	☐	☐
Laugh regularly.	☐	☐
Find ways to make everyday or routine tasks interesting or satisfying.	☐	☐

EMOTIONAL & SPIRITUAL-WELLNESS CONTINUED	Achievement	Satisfaction
Rate your achievement and personal satisfaction with your current wellness.	**Yes, I already do this**	**I would like to change this**
Find times to kick back and relax.	☐	☐
Regularly do things that make you happy.	☐	☐
Celebrate personal accomplishments.	☐	☐
Approach life with honesty.	☐	☐
Explore your talents and interests.	☐	☐
Be open to new ideas and experiences.	☐	☐
Follow through on working toward your goals and dreams.	☐	☐
Be in touch with your inner feelings and motivations.	☐	☐
Develop your own sense of spirituality and meaning in your life.	☐	☐
Find ways to make a contribution to the world.	☐	☐
PHYSICAL WELLNESS	Achievement	Satisfaction
Rate your achievement and personal satisfaction with your current wellness.	**Yes, I already do this**	**I would like to change this**
Keep your body flexible through regular stretching.	☐	☐
Keep your muscles in tone through lifting weights or some sort of resistance workout.	☐	☐
Enjoy at least two forms of physical activity (such as biking, walking or swimming).	☐	☐
Keep your heart fit by taking part in 30 minutes or more of physical activity most days of the week.	☐	☐

PHYSICAL WELLNESS CONTINUED	Achievement	Satisfaction
Rate your achievement and personal satisfaction with your current wellness.	Yes, I already do this	I would like to change this
Not smoke.	☐	☐
Avoid smoky places.	☐	☐
Organize your home and/or work to avoid injury (including such elements as lighting, lifting, and safety gear).	☐	☐
Wear a seat belt at all times when riding in a car.	☐	☐
Never ride in a car that is driven by someone (including yourself) who has been drinking or is driving recklessly.	☐	☐
For men: consume fewer than 12 drinks per week and fewer than 4 drinks on any single occasion, not exceeding 1 drink per hour.	☐	☐
For women: consume fewer than 9 drinks per week and fewer than 3 drinks on any single occasion, not exceeding 1 drink per hour.	☐	☐
Avoid activities that place you at high risk for AIDS (including unprotected sex with multiple partners and sharing needles).	☐	☐
Avoid recreational drug use.	☐	☐
Eat foods that are low in fat.	☐	☐
Eat foods that are high in fiber.	☐	☐
Consume little, if any, caffeine (such as less than 3 cups of coffee).	☐	☐
Avoid eating refined sugar.	☐	☐

PHYSICAL WELLNESS CONTINUED	Achievement	Satisfaction
Rate your achievement and personal satisfaction with your current wellness.	Yes, I already do this	I would like to change this
Be within 10 pounds of your ideal weight.	☐	☐
Brush your teeth at least twice daily.	☐	☐
Floss your teeth daily.	☐	☐
Visit your dentist at least once a year for treatment or a checkup.	☐	☐
Undergo recommended health screenings and physicals.	☐	☐
Have at least one health professional with whom you feel comfortable discussing medical problems.	☐	☐
Research and verify medical recommendations.	☐	☐
Be a careful consumer of medical resources by getting second opinions where appropriate, following through on treatment plans and asking about costs.	☐	☐
ECONOMIC WELLNESS	Achievement	Satisfaction
Rate your achievement and personal satisfaction with your current wellness.	Yes, I already do this	I would like to change this
Sharpen your employment skills through continuing education, reading and discussing your work with others.	☐	☐
Ask for fair compensation for the work you do.	☐	☐

ECONOMIC WELLNESS CONTINUED	Achievement	Satisfaction
Rate your achievement and personal satisfaction with your current wellness.	Yes, I already do this	I would like to change this
Speak up to stop mistreatment of yourself or coworkers.	☐	☐
Join with others in the workplace in eliminating unsafe products and consumer fraud.	☐	☐
Have a detailed personal financial plan that will achieve your short- and long-term goals.	☐	☐
Organize your spending practices so that you live within your means.	☐	☐
Be in agreement about money matters with your spouse or domestic partner.	☐	☐
Comparison shop for the best combination of product, customer service and price.	☐	☐
Avoid materialism (that is, buying because of advertising, sales pressure or just to have what others have).	☐	☐
Make purchases that reflect your personal values.	☐	☐
Save environmental resources and money by fixing and maintaining your possessions, recycling, choosing energy-efficient products, avoiding unnecessary driving and using less energy.	☐	☐
Pay your credit card bills in full and on time.	☐	☐
Pay your rent or mortgage, utilities, taxes and car payments on time.	☐	☐

ECONOMIC WELLNESS CONTINUED	Achievement	Satisfaction
Rate your achievement and personal satisfaction with your current wellness.	**Yes, I already do this**	**I would like to change this**
Have enough financial reserves (not including retirement savings) to last at least 6 months without employment.	☐	☐
Have enough investments or life insurance available in the event of your death to meet the living expenses and tuition of your children until they become adults.	☐	☐
Adequately fund your retirement account or pension.	☐	☐
Be sure you are getting a reasonable rate of return for the investment risks you are taking.	☐	☐
Protect your investments through diversification.	☐	☐
Choose investments that reflect your personal values (such as environmental, social justice and nonviolence).	☐	☐
Have a close friend or family member who would come through for you if you had financial problems.	☐	☐
Be able to help friends and family members with financial problems.	☐	☐
Make contributions to causes and charities that you believe in.	☐	☐

SOCIAL WELLNESS	Achievement	Satisfaction
Rate your achievement and personal satisfaction with your current wellness.	**Yes, I already do this**	**I would like to change this**
Develop, renew and maintain friendships.	☐	☐
Socialize with friends on a regular basis.	☐	☐
Have at least 2 close relationships.	☐	☐
Experience the love and affection you need.	☐	☐
Feel close to your family.	☐	☐
Introduce yourself and greet people you encounter.	☐	☐
Regularly get together with others to play games, enjoy friendly competitions, go to the movies or attend community/cultural events.	☐	☐
Value diversity (appreciate variety in backgrounds and beliefs).	☐	☐
See other people as basically good until proven otherwise.	☐	☐
Respond in others' time of need.	☐	☐
Be a good listener.	☐	☐
Acknowledge your mistakes.	☐	☐
Resolve conflict in positive ways.	☐	☐
Cheer others on.	☐	☐
Share credit for success.	☐	☐
Celebrate the accomplishments of others.	☐	☐
Be honest.	☐	☐
Offer constructive feedback to others in a nonjudgmental way.	☐	☐

SOCIAL WELLNESS CONTINUED	Achievement	Satisfaction
Rate your achievement and personal satisfaction with your current wellness.	**Yes, I already do this**	**I would like to change this**
Feel comfortable in social situations.	☐	☐
Feel comfortable taking a leadership role.	☐	☐
Feel comfortable participating in groups or teams.	☐	☐
Team up well on tasks or projects.	☐	☐
Join a support group when faced with continuing (chronic) physical or emotional problems.	☐	☐

Using Wellness Lifestyle Inventory Results to Become a Better Role Model

There is no good or bad score for the *Wellness Lifestyle Inventory*. Wellness is more about making conscious choices and working toward achieving full potential than it is about meeting a universal standard.

- The boxes you checked in the Achievement column are wellness strengths. Pay special attention to those strengths that correspond to the goals of the current workplace wellness program. Your achievements with these behaviors show that you can "walk the talk" of your wellness program.

- Your wellness goals and your efforts to achieve these goals could be a source of inspiration for employees. Once again, pay special attention to the behaviors that correspond with current workplace wellness program goals. If possible, make a goal that shows your interest in the wellness program.

- Try to use wellness program resources to help achieve your goals. This will show others that participation is worthwhile.

Learning Assignment

Modeling to Reflect the Wellness Program Vision

Develop your plan for making your own conduct consistent with the wellness vision.

What healthy practices are central to the wellness initiative? And how will your conduct become consistent with these practices?

What personal changes, if any, would better reflect the wellness vision?

How might you increase the visibility of your positive practices?

How might you show your willingness to change?

How might you reduce the impact and visibility of your unhealthy behaviors?

How might you show your support for participating in the wellness program?

Demonstrating the Power of Support

In American culture, it is common to approach lifestyle improvement as a private affair. Asking for help tends to be viewed as less desirable and as a show of weakness. However, most of the evidence about what it takes to sustain daily behavior change runs counter to this "go it alone" approach. The greatest likelihood of successful behavior change is achieved when individual initiative is combined with the support of family, friends and coworkers. You can become a role model for this more enlightened approach by actively seeking and acknowledging the support of others. You will also want to prompt employees to offer peer support for healthy lifestyle choices.

The most common form of support is listening. With this form of support, someone agrees to hear about someone else's plans and how they are going. This is a good start, but your wellness program should consider the many additional ways peers and coworkers can play a positive role in supporting one another's lifestyle change efforts. Peers can:

1. **Help refine and clarify wellness goals.** This includes coming up with short-term and long-term goals as well as thinking through how these goals fit within the larger context of overall wellness.

2. **Help find a good role model.** People can learn a lot from someone who has achieved similar goals. You or one of your coworkers could be such a role model, helping others by telling your success story. Coworkers can also put one another in touch with a good role model. This person would be interviewed so the person making the behavior change could learn more about what worked, what challenges were overcome and other tips that might be useful.

3. **Help eliminate or reduce barriers to change.** People usually need time and other resources to achieve their wellness goals. Peers can help coworkers overcome the obstacles that tend to arise during those efforts.

4. **Help find supportive environments.** It is easier to make changes when coworkers are behaving in ways that are consistent with wellness goals. Peers can change their behavior to be a positive influence. They can suggest people and places that will be supportive. They can help coworkers develop strategies for limiting contact with less-supportive environments, and increasing contact with environments that better support wellness goals.

5. **Help avoid relapse and get back on track.** Stressful times and certain locations pose a high risk for reverting to previous unhealthy behavior. Peers can help their coworkers avoid and manage situations that are likely to trigger the old undesired behaviors. They can also be available in times of relapse to offer encouragement and to help others move beyond guilt and toward action.

6. **Help celebrate success and enjoy the rewards.** Most successes go unacknowledged. This is unfortunate, because it is a missed opportunity for some fun and because rewards reinforce behavior change. Peers can help coworkers see the rewards. Peers can reinforce people's efforts by helping them celebrate all along the way to long-term behavior change. Progress and anniversaries can be honored. Coworkers can identify many occasions to celebrate as well as determine the most meaningful way to make successes count.

These six examples of lifestyle change support represent a large and relatively untapped wellness resource. My book, *Healthy Habits, Helpful Friends*, teaches readers about these peer support skills. You may want to consult this book as you pursue opportunities to role model both giving and getting peer support for wellness goals.

You should also find a way to express your enthusiasm for the professional support. Such support is available from personal coaches, counselors, therapists and support group programs such as Weight Watchers and Alcoholics Anonymous. If you have used professional support, consider letting your employees know about your experience. Try to reduce perceived barriers to the use of professional support by stating your openness to scheduling time for such activities.

Learning Assignment
Showing the Power of Support

Develop your plan for showing the value of the support of your friends, family and coworkers.

How will you let people know that you have experienced the benefits of peer support?

How will you model openness to getting support for your own lifestyle goals?

What will you do to inform people about the many ways they can help others achieve wellness?

Modeling Kindness

Your attitude toward wellness will set the tone for others. A spirit of kindness and mutual assistance will go a long way toward nurturing a well workplace culture. You need not be a wellness expert, therapist or counselor to assist. You could, for example, offer words of encouragement. You could respect someone's right to privacy and free choice. You could become a wellness mentor. You could also use your decision-making authority to reduce barriers. You could show appreciation for what others have accomplished. And you could acknowledge those who support the wellness initiative.

As can be seen from this list, there are many ways you can show kindness and thoughtfulness. You are likely to be comfortable with some of these strategies and less comfortable with others. Pick and choose those strategies that seem most appropriate. Try to keep conversations friendly and informal. The best assistance normally comes in the form of good questions. You do not want to tell a coworker what to do. Rather, you want your coworker to decide on the goals and strategies that are best suited to his needs and circumstances. Your offer is to be helpful and to try to create conditions that will give the best chances of success.

Another aspect of kindness is confronting disrespect and unfairness. Too often, wellness has been used in a heavy-handed way to embarrass those with unhealthy lifestyles. For example, people who smoke or are overweight have been ridiculed in an effort to promote change. Some wellness efforts have adopted a "Big Brother" approach, where combinations of sticks and carrots have been used to push people toward change. You can support wellness by challenging those practices that belittle employees or force compliance. You can challenge those approaches that focus attention on people's weaknesses. You can point to a positive and affirming approach that is more consistent with the spirit of wellness and personal empowerment.

Learning Assignment
Showing Kindness

Develop your plan for showing a caring attitude toward wellness.

How will you let people know that you respect their privacy and their right to make their own wellness decisions?

How will people know that you would like to assist in any way you can?

How will you show appreciation for your employees' efforts to support the wellness initiative?

How might you confront disrespect and unfairness that might be occurring?

Serving as an Effective Role Model Checklist

☐ Consider the qualities of effective role models. Are there ways you could improve in these areas? How will you tone down or eliminate attitudes that may undermine your effectiveness?

☐ Conduct a strength review of your own wellness practices (The *Wellness Lifestyle Inventory* could be used for this purpose). How will you make these positive practices more visible to your coworkers?

☐ Determine your opportunities for lifestyle improvement. Pay particular attention to those behaviors that are now being emphasized in your organization's wellness program. Are you willing to change some or all of these unhealthy behaviors? If yes, how will employees know of your interest in making such a change? If no, how will you reduce the visibility of your unhealthy practices?

☐ Examine all the opportunities to participate in the wellness program. How will you visibly participate in a way that might inspire the participation of other employees?

☐ Take stock of your support network for achieving your own healthy lifestyle goals. How will you acknowledge the support you are receiving? How will you engage more people in supporting your lifestyle improvement efforts?

☐ Examine how you can show kindness and mutual respect through your efforts to promote wellness. How can you increase your capacity to show these qualities? How might you help reduce any unfairness, undue control, or disrespect being experienced as a result of the wellness initiative?

Leadership Stories

◆ Jolene recognized that she could become a better role model. She never stopped for lunch and rarely left the office before 6:00. She liked being praised for her dedication, but she needed to find another way to show her commitment to the company. She decided to put work/life balance on the agenda of the next staff meeting. The discussion quickly turned to working smarter rather than harder. Her staff agreed that longer hours sometimes meant less mental focus and energy. Jolene committed to taking walks during the noon hour. She also committed to being out the door by 5:30. Her staff joined in with their own work/life balance goals.

◆ At first Rick didn't really think he had much to offer in terms of being a wellness role model. His weight was creeping up, and his days on the sports field seemed far away. Rick completed the Wellness Lifestyle Inventory. To his surprise, he found he had many positive practices, particularly in the areas of emotional, social and economic wellness. The results helped him see many strengths. Maybe he could be a role model after all.

◆ Flo knew that her people wouldn't go unless she took the lead. She signed up for a lunchtime walking group and let everyone know about her plan. This really broke the ice. The majority of her staff signed up for something. Best of all, the attention spawned a workplace support network for Flo. People get her out the door and moving by noon.

◆ Chan decided to become less of a negative role model. He declared that he would light up only away from work. He also would no longer drag his people out for a drink. The next staff outing would be something healthier. Golfing or hiking seemed like more fun anyway.

◆ Acacia enjoys being helpful, and wellness is one more way to reach out. She particularly likes coming up with work-arounds for time and money conflicts. Her wellness motto, "Let's do it," is a variation on the old Nike tag line, "Just do it." Acacia likes her social approach better. "Just do it" sounded so lonely.

Chapter 4: Aligning Cultural Touch Points

In "Creating a Shared Wellness Vision," you established wellness norm goals. These goals set forth behaviors that will become the new "way we do things around here." This chapter, "Aligning Cultural Touch Points," is about adjusting rewards, modeling, communication and other environmental features so that they reinforce and do not impede desired wellness behavior.

Cultural touch points are similar to a spider's web. Many strands of this cultural web of influence are visible and written in policy. For example, smoking policies are posted in plain sight. Such formal policies help many nonsmokers avoid secondhand smoke and have encouraged many smokers to quit. Other strands in the web of cultures are less visible and become apparent only when they are pressed into action. For example, we are likely to be less aware of the subculture of friendship that has formed among smokers in designated smoking areas. The social bonds between smokers are a less visible aspect of the culture. This social network makes it difficult to quit smoking.

Achieving wellness norm goals requires examining the web of influences and then making strategic adjustments. Cultural touch points represent strategic leadership opportunities for shaping the culture's influence on people. Descriptions of 10 cultural touch points follow.

Rewards and Recognition

When it comes to rewards, financial incentives often receive the most attention. Rewards also come in the form of praise, increased autonomy, first choice on job responsibilities, access to resources and promotion. Leaders can fine-tune the various systems of rewards so that they are more consistent with wellness norm goals. The goal is for employees to report that people in their work group are rewarded and recognized for healthy lifestyle choices.

Reward systems are already in place in most workplace cultures. Your wellness leadership responsibility is to identify these systems and align them with wellness goals. The following illustrations show some of the likely possibilities.

- Wellness could be given consideration in a performance appraisal.

- A wellness philosophy could be one of the selection criteria for promotions.

- The bonus system could include wellness goals.

- Holiday gatherings and events could celebrate wellness practices.

Reduce or eliminate rewards for unhealthy practices. For example, it might be common to praise employees for working through lunch or for working late. A healthier approach would be to acknowledge people who find a way to get work done without undermining their work breaks or life outside of work.

Leaders can also adjust the types of rewards to be consistent with a wellness message. High-calorie foods such as cakes have been typical rewards. Healthier and equally celebratory foods need to replace such rewards. Another example is giving time off from work, which sends an unintended message that work is somehow undesirable. A new approach would be to offer subsidies for vacations of a healthier nature. As can be seen in these examples, finding healthier rewards could amplify the positive impact of reward systems.

Make it clear that wellness program rewards are available in addition to the natural benefits of healthy living. Many quality-of-life benefits and reduced costs are the automatic result of lifestyle improvements. Such benefits are called "intrinsic rewards." For example, an ex-smoker immediately cuts her cost of cigarettes and reduces the likelihood of getting a cold. "Extrinsic rewards" are extra benefits that are available from the organization. When we give an extrinsic reward such as lowered insurance costs we are adding to the intrinsic rewards. It is helpful to point out that both types of benefits are available through achieving wellness goals.

You can adjust rewards to make sure they are meaningful to your employees. Some employees would want their efforts to remain private. You can see to it that these rewards are handled in a confidential way. Some employees would appreciate public acknowledgment and celebration. You can make sure that appropriate levels of fanfare and acclaim are provided. And you can pick rewards so that they hit the mark. Some employees would appreciate money; others want a non-cash prize.

Some of the most powerful rewards honor group achievements. Team sports often result in such collective rewards. This approach can be extended to work teams and to a variety of wellness goals. If two people accomplish a goal together, this should be acknowledged. If someone plays a special role in reducing barriers to wellness at the worksite, this should be recognized. If a whole work group joins together to achieve a wellness goal, find a way to express your appreciation. The chances are good that goals achieved with others will make a lasting impression.

> ## Learning Assignment
> ## Aligning Rewards and Recognition
>
> Examine opportunities for using rewards and recognition to reinforce new wellness norms.
>
> How will existing reward systems be modified to better support wellness practices?
>
> How will the current rewards for undesired behavior be reduced or eliminated?
>
> What new reward and recognition initiatives will be introduced?
>
> How will the choice of rewards change so they are more consistent with wellness?
>
> How will wellness rewards be adjusted to reflect desired levels of personal privacy and public acclaim?
>
> How will groups and teams be rewarded and recognized for their collective wellness efforts?

Push-back

We often think of push-back in terms of how we will stop people from doing the wrong thing. For example, no-smoking policies are a way to confront smoking behavior. Seat belt laws and safety rules use confrontation to promote healthier practices. Policies that restrict the use of alcohol and other drugs are additional examples. You have a role in reinforcing these rules. You can:

- Remind people of these rules. Hopefully, your entire work group will cooperate with friendly reminders so that more drastic measures are not required.

- Enforce the rules. Consistent, timely and direct feedback sends a clear message.

- Make sure that support is available for required changes. No-smoking policies, for example, are better received when employees are given a warning period and provided medical and group support for quitting.

A second, and frequently overlooked, dimension of push-back occurs when healthy practices are confronted. For example, someone who meditates at work is likely to be told that his or her behavior is out of place. Resistance may also be felt by people who are more careful in their food choices, who exercise regularly or who stretch during the workday. Driving at the speed limit might be called old-fashioned. Taking safety precautions and getting regular health screenings may earn someone the label of a worrywart and hypochondriac. You can reduce the level of confrontation for positive practices if you:

- Praise healthy practices that are being confronted. You can further reinforce this action by rewarding and recognizing the employee for taking on such an unpopular lifestyle practice.

- Remove any policy disincentives. For example, if health screening is to become the norm, the cost of it should be picked up by health insurance.

- Ask your employees to refrain from being critical of healthy practices. Many employees do not even realize that they are confronting healthy behavior. They may be willing to endorse healthy practices, or at very least let it go.

> **Learning Assignment**
> **Aligning Push-back**
>
> Examine opportunities to confront unhealthy practices and reduce the push-back against healthy practices.
>
> How can unhealthy practices best be confronted?
>
> What will be done to reduce the counterproductive push-back against desired wellness practices?

Relationships

Most people will stick with wellness activities that maintain positive relationships. We are more likely to try new activities if they will help us make new friends, find a mate or expand our professional networks. The hope for a powerful ally or mentor is yet another example of the influence of relationships. We tend to continue behaviors that include our friends and close colleagues.

Reference groups are another example of how relationships influence behavior. Unions and professional associations are examples of such reference groups. We tend to avoid activities that make us feel out of step. We tend to act in ways that help us fit in with our group.

People often think of relationships as something that undermines wellness goals. Such would be the case in considering relationships with drinking buddies and smoking buddies and when thinking about the unhealthy food customarily served at social occasions. When thinking about aligning this touch point, try to reduce these negative associations while increasing positive social opportunities.

Relationships can work for wellness goals. You can steer your employees toward participating in wellness activities together. You can also incorporate a social component into wellness activities. And you can advocate for making wellness activities available to friends, housemates and family.

Peer support is a powerful and frequently underutilized tool for wellness. Most people do not have adequate training in how to give or get support for lifestyle improvement. In addition to listening and offering words of encouragement, peers can help set goals, identify role models, eliminate barriers to change, locate supportive environments, work through relapse and celebrate success. Some organizations are training peer mentors to enhance the quantity and quality of peer support. Information about such programs is available in the book *Healthy Habits, Helpful Friends* and online at www.wellnessmentor.net. You could encourage such a peer support initiative at your workplace. If one is already in place, you could encourage participation.

Relationships also make wellness activities more enjoyable. Mealtime could be an occasion to enjoy healthy foods in the company of others. In addition, outdoor adventure activities, sports, picnics, spa programs, conferences, support groups and classes can mix healthy lifestyles and social engagement.

Learning Assignment
Aligning Relationships

Examine opportunities for building friendships, work teams, professional networks and other positive relationships in conjunction with wellness behavior.

How can the positive wellness behavior be integrated into social activities or have a stronger social component?

How can unhealthy practices become disengaged from positive social outcomes?

How can peer support be mobilized for wellness goals?

Modeling

We examined many aspects of modeling in "Serving as an Effective Role Model." You can extend this idea by helping develop other workplace role models. This will add to the diversity and availability of wellness role models. For example, you may not have smoked, but you may be able to identify someone who has successfully quit. If willing, this person could serve as a role model to those who would like to quit. He could explain what was accomplished and how.

Your goal is to increase the visibility and availability of wellness role models. Start with behaviors that are currently being emphasized in your wellness program. For example, if your wellness norm goals are for physical activity, let it be known that you are interested in fitness activities. Listen for inspirational stories. You want role models who are respected and admired within your work group. You can further screen your candidates by picking people who already have the qualities of effective role models. These were listed in the "Serving as an Effective Role Model" chapter. Once you have identified someone who might make a good role model, ask whether she is willing to make her efforts public. Your role models must be open to public disclosure.

Many past wellness program participants are likely to be great role model candidates. These participants tend to be enthusiastic about what they have accomplished, and they are likely to want to share their enthusiasm with those contemplating change. They can give firsthand accounts of their efforts and what was achieved. Personal testimonials from peers can have a powerful impact.

Don't forget stories about what workplaces and work groups have achieved. Well workplaces make good role models too. They show what can be accomplished when people pull together to promote wellness. You are may already know stories of particularly successful work groups and organizations. Wellness professionals, books, magazines and Web sites are also sources for such success stories. Local, state and national well workplace awards programs are additional good sources for identifying successful organizations. There is likely to be a healthy workplace awards program in your state.

Learning Assignment
Aligning Modeling

Examine opportunities for using role modeling to reinforce new wellness norms.

How will you identify qualified employees who are willing to serve as wellness role models?

How will you identify work groups and organizations with wellness stories that will inspire your work group?

How will you take advantage of early successes to create new role models?

How will you spread the word about the individual and work group role models you have identified?

Recruitment and Selection

Unhealthy groups draw less health-oriented individuals. An example of this is when a college is listed in magazines as a "party school." The incoming class is likely to be looking to party. Your work group should gain a reputation for being a well workplace. This will attract candidates who are open to healthy lifestyles. Just as winning sports teams find it easier to recruit the most promising athletes, you will find it easier to draw health-oriented people to your group.

You can actively recruit and select new team members who

are open to wellness. A wellness statement could be incorporated into an announcement for the position. The benefits of employment could be expressed in a way that highlights wellness activities. Prospects could be asked about their current wellness interests and activities. Those prospects who show enthusiasm for wellness could be encouraged to pursue the position.

Learning Assignment
Aligning Recruitment and Selection

Examine opportunities for using the employee recruitment and selection process to establish and maintain wellness norms.

What will you do to get a reputation for wellness?

How will you make your well workplace culture visible to prospective employees?

How will you encourage wellness-oriented prospects to pursue employment in your work group?

First Impressions

Employees' early experiences make a strong impression. It is an all-too-common mistake to neglect wellness in the haste to get a new employee working. A new hire quickly determines whether healthy food choices or fitness activities will be accepted in his or her work group. The first meal in the cafeteria or break room speaks volumes about whether healthy eating is a priority. Informal conversations and the first night out with coworkers could overwhelm any positive messages that are offered by the wellness program. You don't want your new people to get the false impression that unhealthy practices are common or that there is little concern about wellness. See to it that getting people off to a healthy start with the right first impression is a high priority.

You can ensure that employees' early impressions are positive ones by explaining the wellness vision and how they can participate in wellness activities, including connecting them with wellness role models. Wellness lifestyle assessments and feedback could also be a part of the orientation process.

Some organizations are incorporating wellness mentoring into the orientation process. A new employee is paired up with a veteran for mutual support in the pursuit of healthy lifestyle goals. The mentoring relationship is supported by peer support training offered as part of the orientation program or in an online format. The resulting early friendship helps create a positive peer culture. Further information about this approach is available at www.well-nessmentor.net or in *Healthy Habits, Helpful Friends*.

Learning Assignment
Aligning First Impressions

Examine opportunities for using the orientation experiences of new employees to establish and maintain wellness norms.

How will your new employees become aware of wellness goals and initiatives?

How will new employees avoid getting the wrong first impression that unhealthy practices are normal?

How will new hires build friendships and professional networks through healthy lifestyle activities?

Learning and Training

People tend to do things they are good at. This simple premise works for and against wellness. If people share skills for how to work without sleep, you are likely to have a fatigued workforce. If, in contrast, people are skilled at yoga, you are likely to see fewer muscular skeletal injuries and more stretching activity. Curtail unhealthy training and encourage training for healthy lifestyles. Where possible, give your employees opportunities to share what they have learned with their work group.

Training is particularly important and powerful when the broader culture is having difficulty with a positive health practice. So, for example, Americans need special training in how to eat healthier on the road or how to select healthier alternatives in the grocery store. American culture makes healthy eating difficult. More training is required for success.

See to it that people get the skills needed to achieve their wellness goals. Keep a list of possible training resources and become familiar with how to access additional options. The Internet, books and self-help guides are ready resources for these skills. Wellness classes may be available at your worksite. If not, consider organizing such classes. Other classes are available in the community. Support groups such as Weight Watchers have an education and training component. Coaches and instructors can be hired for a more personalized educational experience. These services are offered in a variety of convenient formats, including in person, over the telephone and by e-mail.

Learning Assignment
Aligning Learning and Training

Examine opportunities for using training to establish and maintain healthy behaviors.

How will your employees learn skills needed to achieve the goals set forth in your wellness initiative?

How will you curtail training that runs counter to wellness?

Information and Communication

Employees need current, timely, relevant and accurate information. Ideally, this information can be tailored to employees' wellness needs and interests. It should include motivational information about why wellness goals are worthy of commitment, as well as information about what resources are available for pursuing wellness goals.

Unfortunately, in many organizations wellness slips off the radar. The results of surveys are not discussed or acted upon. Commitments to wellness goals go unannounced. Little is known about how people have overcome their wellness obstacles. Wellness program information becomes dated or inaccurate. The fact is that keeping healthy lifestyle changes in focus requires ongoing communication and feedback. Your enthusiastic endorsement of wellness activities can go a long way toward getting people engaged.

You need to use both formal and informal communication mechanisms. It is common for one or more employees to take on the role of being the information clearinghouse. These people would be the best choice for sharing the wellness message through the grapevine. There are many communication options, including e-mail, print and team meetings.

Most communication about health is unnecessarily negative. Keep wellness communication positive, affirming and fun. For example, it is better to talk about lifestyle assets than health risks. We want to take a positive approach by building on people's strengths. Similarly, it is better to discuss the likely benefits we can achieve than it is to scare people about the future. Fear is an attention getter, but it carries an underlying message of desperation. Humor is a great way to communicate. Many aspects of unhealthy behavior are truly ridiculous. An unhealthy culture has gotten us into predicaments that look unnatural and funny. When engaging in humor, be careful not to make fun of individuals. There are plenty of opportunities to make fun of our personal challenges or to jest about the crazy world we live in.

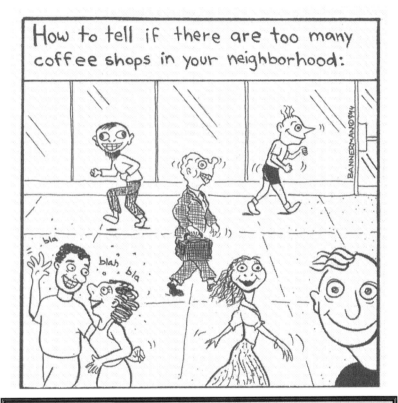

Learning Assignment
Aligning Communication

Examine opportunities for using information and communication to establish and maintain wellness norms.

What information and feedback will be particularly useful for promoting wellness in your work group?

How will individuals and teams get the feedback they need to stay on track?

How will people be kept abreast of new wellness initiatives?

Traditions and Symbols

There is something wonderful about a symbolic act in that it represents much more than first meets the eye. For example, a fitness center can be symbolic of an organization's commitment to wellness. Release time for wellness activities not only helps eliminate a barrier to participation, but also symbolically represents the priority being given to wellness. These are grand gestures. Other, simpler symbols can be created in the form of water bottles, T-shirts, pedometers and other wellness paraphernalia. You can support wellness by coming up with one or more objects, actions or resources that could symbolize the culture's support for healthy lifestyles.

Like symbols, rituals have an influence that go beyond first appearances. For instance, a group of workers could stretch for a couple of minutes before beginning work. This simple act of stretching would soon become a common wellness bond between employees. Other rituals can be seasonal. The annual 5K fun run/walk, the New Year's health resolution and the company picnic are rituals. Similarly, you could make it an annual ritual to complete the health survey. You could transition the office birthday celebration to an occasion for personal reflection, new health commitments and healthy dining. A favorite healthy meal can augment or replace less-healthy traditions. When rituals are changed, wellness can become integrated into the routine.

The transitions of life and work can also be connected to wellness. The trick is to honor such rites of passage with a wellness activity. A new employee can be welcomed with a wellness retreat. The birth of an employee's child can be celebrated with health-oriented gifts. The anniversary of the organization can be acknowledged with a wellness activity. Promotions and retirements can also be connected to wellness activities.

> ### Learning Assignment
> ### Aligning Traditions and Symbols
>
> Examine opportunities for using rites, rituals and symbols to establish and maintain wellness norms.
>
> What is being said about wellness in current traditions and symbols? What can be done to modify these to reflect wellness goals?
>
> What grand gestures and small acts will be symbolic of wellness commitment?
>
> What wellness-related traditions can be added to the workday or calendar?
>
> How will transitions carry a wellness message?

Resource Commitment

The 10th and final cultural touch point involves the commitment of resources. One of the prevailing—and destructive—myths about wellness is that it can or should be done on the cheap. Wellness is a good investment, worthy of time, space and other resources. Help ensure that employees have the wherewithal to succeed. It is far better for people to get the time, equipment, training and other resources they need to achieve wellness goals in grand style. For example, many wellness activities take time. Don't be fooled into thinking that a 15-minute exercise break is just as good as a 45-minute workout. Goofy shortcuts only diminish people's enthusiasm and show that wellness is a low priority. Sometimes wellness involves the commitment of resources. Advocate for these resources.

A primary objective of a wellness program should be to make a wellness lifestyle easier to accomplish. Your employees are likely to have a list of barriers to any wellness goal. Your role is to remove the barriers and to empower people. Until you address one or more of the major barriers, you and your organization will be perceived as less than committed. Show some generosity, creativity and thoughtfulness in reducing these barriers. Your investment will be matched in personal commitment. Your wellness program will no longer be viewed as lip service or wishful thinking.

Enlist the support of your work team and other wellness champions to break down barriers. Maybe an on-site health club is not financially viable, but discounts and subsidies at local private health clubs may be an option. Maybe there is no time in the work schedule for healthy activities—could work breaks be reconfigured to serve this purpose? Perhaps child care and transportation issues could be resolved so that employees have the ability to participate in wellness activities. Maybe wellness activities could be redesigned so that family and friends can participate. Could bikes and bike paths be provided and maintained? A shower installed in an underutilized bathroom? Perhaps area farmers would find it profitable to set up a farmers' market in your parking lot. There are many creative solutions. Many of these actions engender a great sense of pride and ownership in the wellness program.

Learning Assignment
Aligning Resource Commitment

Examine how resources such as time, equipment, space and money can support wellness.

What are the primary resource barriers that might stand in the way of wellness behavior?

How will barriers be reduced or eliminated, making it easier to practice healthy lifestyles?

How will the use of resources show your team that a well workplace is a priority?

Organizing Your Efforts

Changing norms with cultural touch points almost always requires strategic planning. The following principles are useful in devising the most efficient and powerful strategy:

- Use interviews with key decision makers and a cross-section of employees to identify existing strengths and opportunities for improvement. Their input will increase buy-in. Use your interviews to brainstorm a comprehensive list of actions. Also ask about the best ways to carry out the change initiatives. For example, employees could share the best mechanism for implementing a new financial reward program so that it will avoid being perceived as a bribe or as unfair.

- Consult those most affected by changes in cultural touch points. People are much more resistant to changes that are being imposed on them without their consent and involvement. Empowerment is a principle of wellness and should be taken into consideration in any culture change effort. You are trying to engage people in creating a culture they want and need. This is not an effort to manipulate people. Transparency and involvement are keys to successful culture change. Your employees are likely to want a culture that doesn't interfere with their efforts to adopt healthier lifestyles.

- Senior management, union leaders and skilled professionals tend to have the most power to address touch points. They often control the money, written policies, time and other resources. These key decision makers should be engaged in addressing cultural touch points. They are likely to understand that building the corporate culture is an important leadership responsibility. At the very least, they should be informed about plans and progress.

- Share this assignment with other wellness champions. This will make the effort more manageable and will increase the likelihood that you will have a lasting impact on the culture. It is best to work with those people who have a history of getting things done in your workplace. Their political skills and wisdom will be an important asset.

- Build on existing strengths and past efforts. This will make it less likely that you will undermine existing positive influences. Also, it is more appealing to recognize what is going right. Don't overlook past efforts, even if they were insufficient to change the culture.

- Touch points already function in a culture. An all-too-common approach is to try to invent entirely new programs rather than modifying existing and better-established systems. The current system must be adjusted, not replaced. For example, try to work with existing communication, rewards and training programs. Pick just a couple of highly visible and necessary activities to add to the mix. You may, for instance, find that there are no current rituals that support the desired wellness behavior. You could fill the gap by adding a daily or yearly ritual.

- Address more than enough touch points to tip the balance toward wellness. This tipping point can be reached only when enough influences support desired behavior. Using only one or two touch points often results in unintended and negative consequences. Think of your efforts in terms of changing the web of influences. You can yank at one strand of the web, but it is likely to make a mess of the culture. You need to strengthen some aspects of the web and weaken others. Such coordinated action will shift the culture with less disruption and resistance.

Learning Assignment

Organize Your Efforts to Align Touch Points

Draw from the ideas you have developed for each touch point and develop an overall plan of action. Your strategic plan will address the following questions:

What research is needed to get a clear picture of how the touch points are influencing key behavior?

What aspects of the cultural touch points support desired behavior? How can these positive influences be reinforced?

What influences undermine or interfere with desired behavior? How can these be eliminated or reduced?

Who will be most affected by change and how will they be involved in the effort?

How will you involve key decision makers in the process of changing the touch points?

What group of influences will be modified to reach a tipping point?

Aligning Cultural Touch Points Checklist

Address the touch points:

☐ What will be done about creating effective role models?

☐ What will be done about rewarding and recognizing desired behavior?

☐ What will be done about reducing negative push-back and increasing desired push-back?

☐ What new training will be available and how will counter-productive learning be reduced?

☐ How will you recruit and select people who are open to wellness goals?

☐ How will new employees get a good first impression of the wellness effort?

☐ What will be communicated about wellness behavior?

☐ How will people form positive relationships around desired behavior rather than unhealthy behavior?

☐ What will be done to adjust and create traditions, rituals and symbols to reflect desired behavior?

☐ How will the use of resources such as time, space and money demonstrate a commitment to desired wellness behavior?

☐ Develop a plan for efficiently working with cultural touch points. Have you taken full advantage of cultural strengths and all change options? What list of touch point changes will achieve the tipping point? Have you addressed the touch points that are the best leverage points for norm goals?

☐ Consider the authority needed to modify cultural touch points. Which wellness champions need to be engaged in addressing touch points? Do these people have a track record of bringing about change? Do these champions have enough political power to make the change happen?

☐ Examine your approach to involvement. How will your employees have input? What will you do to help employees take ownership and responsibility for making the changes work?

Case Stories

◆ Alonzo knew his team was on edge. The last layoff had left everyone dispirited. He hoped the market would turn around. Alonzo decided to use the touch points as a framework for making the shift to a positive culture. Each month one or two touch points would be given special consideration. The focus on communication had already paid off. The rumor mill was being replaced by a humor mill. His door was covered with favorite cartoons. Next month there would be a seminar on positive psychology. It would be interesting to see how training would feed into the culture shift.

◆ Too many fatal accidents put alcohol abuse on Sarah's agenda. This time the response had to go beyond another seminar and bigger penalties. The safety teams identified a menu of bold steps. Families would be involved in a new education initiative. Employees were to receive training in how to recognize and handle substance abuse at work. A mental health hotline would be established and counselors were to be available on-site. All company-sponsored activities were going alcohol free. The company was also going to sponsor longer hours for on-site restaurants and health clubs. Evening and night shift workers were to have alternatives to the bars.

◆ The Benson Company set a goal to achieve national objectives for physical activity, healthy eating and nonsmoking. Focus interviews were held at each worksite and on every shift. The 10 touch points were the subject. Employees identified many strategies for culture change. Each worksite, work group and shift had its own list. Management took the lead in implementing strategies for each lifestyle objective.

◆ National smoking rates were among the highest in the world. The researchers identified a message that really cut deep into the culture. Everyone loved children. People would respond to information about the negative impact of secondhand smoke on children. The public health ads were run with information about how to enroll in free smoking cessation programs. Hospitals, schools and major employers were implementing restrictive smoking policies. A total ban on cigarette advertising would soon be in place.

◆ So far confederated bank's goal of having their employees become careful consumers of medical resources seemed like a joke. Price lists were unavailable and the health care providers were clueless about the cost of their own services. The providers insisted it would be difficult to offer pricing because each insurance carrier had negotiated different prices. In addition, employees reported that any talk of money seemed to be embarrassing and out of place. The human resources director formed an advisory group to look at cultural influences.

Chapter 5: Monitoring and Celebrating Success

Monitoring and celebrating are important wellness leadership functions. Consider the impact:

- Ongoing attention shows that these efforts are being taken seriously.

- Keeping track and offering constructive feedback make it possible to fine-tune wellness efforts.

- Thoughtfulness in selecting meaningful and appropriate ways to honor progress shows that you really care.

Both monitoring and celebrating wellness require a positive behavioral approach. Your efforts should be multifaceted, relying on physical tests, observation, focus interviews and self-report. These metrics must be tailored to the traditions and mind-sets of your work culture. You will complete the feedback loop by seeing to it that new information leads to praise, celebration and program adjustments. And you must work to break free of old negative patterns of pointing fingers, finding fault and appealing to fear. Effective wellness program feedback is strength building and inspiring.

Creating a Wellness Dashboard

Those who design cars and planes pay careful attention to the dashboard. The beauty of a good dashboard is that it puts key information at your fingertips without distracting you from your primary driving task. A wellness dashboard should have a similar design. You need ready and convenient information prepared in such a way that it doesn't distract you from your other management responsibilities.

Narrow your data collection to actionable information. Some organizations have mistakenly made the *collection* of information primary and the use of that information secondary. The medical system generates a nearly endless supply of numbers. It all sounds important until you realize that unless underlying behavior is changed, little should be expected from tracking illnesses, treatments and their associated costs. Our highly complicated medical care system makes it easy to spend more on measuring employee health and productivity than on actually assisting employees in their lifestyle improvement efforts. You want enough information to drive your wellness program, but not so much information that you get lost in the details. Your information should be purposeful and should make it possible to celebrate accomplishments in a timely fashion. Your dashboard must also be organized so that you can make proper adjustments before your group loses enthusiasm and focus.

Organize your wellness dashboard so that it tracks performance, programmatic results and cultural results. Performance measures are the bottom-line indicators of success; they include health behavior, productivity and illness costs. Programmatic measures assess the degree to which the program is reaching and engaging your people. Cultural measures determine the extent to which the environment supports positive practices and discourages unhealthy behavior. Taken together, these three broad categories offer a complete picture of organizational wellness.

Performance Measures: What Counts?

Most wellness activities are directed at healthy lifestyles. The purpose is to help people adopt new health behaviors and to avoid unhealthy practices. Progress in achieving desired behavior will depend on the answer to the four questions below.

1. **What percentage of your people are currently engaged in the wellness behavior?** From this figure you can determine how many people could benefit from change. Hopefully, many employees have already achieved the desired behavior. These employees model the positive practice for others.

2. **What is the rate of lifestyle change attempts?** Your goal is to motivate those with unhealthy practices to try to change. You can ask employees if they have recently attempted to change a health practice. Fortunately, most employees make one or more such attempts annually.

3. **What is the lifestyle change success rate?** Your goal is to drive up lasting and positive behavior change. You can ask employees to rate their success. The gold standard for most behavior changes is that the healthy practice has been maintained for six months or longer.

4. **What percentage of your people are adopting un-healthy practices?** For example, despite your wellness initiative, some formerly physically active employees may stop exercising. In this example, you would ask employees if they have become less active. Your goal is to create conditions that prevent employees from abandoning their positive practices.

Wellness behaviors can be counted through self-report, observation and physical tests. A list of sample health practices questions used for self-report is provided in Appendix A. The type of measurement depends on the behavior. If, for example, your goal is to promote physical fitness, self-reports of weekly physical activity can be combined with physiological measures of cardiovascular health, strength, flexibility and agility. Fitness center and walking path utilization rates could add to the overall picture.

Maintaining privacy and confidentiality is very important. For this reason, it is recommended that you either collect this data anonymously or have a wellness company conduct an independent assessment. You are interested in aggregate, not personal, information. Your efforts to keep information private will increase the accuracy of employee responses. Maintaining privacy also reduces the likelihood of violating legal safeguards.

Collect your data in such a way that it will be easy to assess progress and to set team goals. Behavior should be assessed at least annually. Typically, the information is collected by a health coach or as part of an annual employee health survey. To achieve optimal participation, establish a week on the calendar for measurement and a date soon thereafter for celebrating progress. Try to turn your efforts to monitor and celebrate success into a positive annual ritual. You can, for instance, coordinate this effort with New Year's celebrations and resolutions.

Secondary Performance Measures

In addition to measuring health behavior, many organizations develop a second bottom line that corresponds with the wellness benefits. Examples include medical cost savings, productivity increases, enhanced health, improved public goodwill, heightened morale and a decrease in accidents. The following list of benefits and measurement strategies are examples of such bottom-line indicators.

Wellness Benefits and Measures

Wellness Program Benefit	Measurement Strategies
Longer, healthier and happier lives associated with achieving healthier lifestyles.	Health practices questionnaires, also known as health risk appraisals (see a sample at www.realage.com).
Cost savings through decreased need for medical care, speedier recoveries and better management of chronic conditions.	Review of accident or injury rates, medical costs and disability claims.
Improved productivity through improved work readiness, lowered absenteeism and reduced turnover.	Review of job performance, absenteeism and turnover data. It is also possible to survey employees about how their mental and physical health influences their work.
Better morale and teamwork through the fun, mutual support and kindness engendered through wellness activities.	Employee morale, teamwork and work satisfaction surveys.
Enhanced organizational image that is associated with treating employees well.	Public opinion surveys, marketing data and measures of favorable press.

Unfortunately, many of these wellness benefits are difficult and expensive to track. There are a lot of complicating factors that have nothing to do with the wellness effort. For example, your wellness program cannot be held accountable for a flu epidemic or for skyrocketing drug prices. Morale is often influenced by management style and by current economic conditions. These are just some of the complicating factors that make it difficult to prove that the wellness program has made a difference. Fortunately, the *American Journal of Health Promotion* (www.healthpromotionjournal.com) and other research publications regularly report the findings of studies designed to rigorously test the benefits of wellness programs. A review of this literature is likely to reveal stories, best practices and research findings that are relevant to your work group's wellness efforts. Financial forecasting software is now available that attempts to combine your company's available health data with historical averages to predict return on investment (ROI). Health Improvement Solutions (www.healthimprovementsolutions.com) is a source for such an ROI analysis. You may also seek out the assistance of an academic institution or consulting company in developing your own internal research project. One such academic partner is the University of Michigan's Health Management Research Center (www.hmrc.umich.edu).

Several less-complicated and less-expensive strategies are available for assessing the benefits of wellness activities. Although these strategies won't prove anything, they help build the business case. Although imperfect, these approaches are likely to exceed the quality of data that is collected to justify comparable business investments.

Start with the information that is already easily available. Some likely candidates are insurance costs, medical care use rates, absenteeism rates, disability claims and any measure you now use for job performance. Look at trends in this data. Did these trends change with the introduction of wellness programs? Positive trends of this nature support the value of your wellness efforts. Don't be surprised if some people question whether your wellness efforts had anything to do with the business outcomes. Correlation is not the same thing as causation. There are likely to be a number of alternatives that could explain your findings.

Another strategy is to use data from published research to estimate the value of lifestyle change. Such estimates rely upon research reports on the economic value of healthy practices such as physical activity. Reports on the additional cost of unhealthy behavior are also published regularly. For example, a Health

Enhancement Research Organization (HERO) study of more than 46,000 employees found that medical care for obese employees cost 21 percent more, care for smokers cost 20 percent more and care for physically inactive employees cost 10 percent more. Using the HERO data, you can calculate potential lifestyle savings by combining per-person health insurance costs with the number of employees in your work group who have the unhealthy conditions and practices noted above.

A low-cost strategy for forecasting potential economic savings would be to search the scientific literature or to conduct an online search for the most relevant and current data for your program's wellness goals. Keep in mind that most of these estimates are based on averages in a particular population at a particular time. When using your estimates, be sure not to overstate your confidence in the accuracy of your financial forecast. It would be prudent to report on some of the reasons your organization's results could differ.

Learning Assignment

Developing Performance Measures

Your wellness dashboard should achieve quantifiable results in terms of behavior change and wellness benefits such as economic savings and improved productivity.

What health behaviors will be measured and how?

What wellness benefits do you want your employees to achieve and how will you determine if they are getting these benefits?

Programmatic Measures: What's Happening?

Another section of your wellness dashboard should be reserved for programmatic measures. You need to know what is being done and understand the quality of those experiences. At the simplest level, programmatic measures include participation rates and program satisfaction. Answers to the following questions are useful in establishing such programmatic measures.

1. **What is the participation rate for those activities meant for all employees?** Typically, these core activities include completion of a health questionnaire and participation in wellness coaching sessions. This data could include feedback on who has participated and whether or not participants have completed the activity. Your goal is to have a high proportion of employees participate.

2. **What is the participation rate for optional wellness activities?** Typically, these activities include peer support programs, wellness courses, special events, sports activities, wellness games and challenges, and utilization of health information resources. You will set participation goals based on the activity and how it matches your employees' interests.

3. **What is the level of satisfaction with wellness initiatives?** Your employees will rate their program experience. The feedback could be collected through informal conversations or through participant evaluations. Ask about the quality of the program delivery as well as about the program content and format. A second strategy is to ask about past program experience in an annual needs and interest survey. A sample evaluation is provided in Appendix A. Your goal is to have high-quality wellness initiatives that match the needs of your employees.

Learning Assignment

Developing Programmatic Measures

Your wellness dashboard should show that the initiative is reaching your employees and delivering high-quality results.

What primary wellness activities and initiatives will you be tracking?

How will you monitor participation rates?

How will you assess program mix in terms of the availability of wellness offerings and how well they match the needs of your employees?

How will you assess the quality of the wellness activities and participant satisfaction?

Cultural Measures: Is the Environment Supportive?

The culture concept was introduced in the opening chapter, "A Call to Wellness Leadership." The word *culture* originated from the concept of cultivation. Just like good farming practice, wellness leadership creates fertile ground for healthy practices. Five overlapping cultural dimensions—shared values, norms, touch points, peer support and climate—work together to shape behavior. Addressing these cultural dimensions is an underlying theme throughout *Wellness Leadership*. A gauge on your wellness dashboard should show progress in creating a supportive culture. Let's embark on a substantial description of these five dimensions and then tackle how to measure them.

Cultural Dimensions

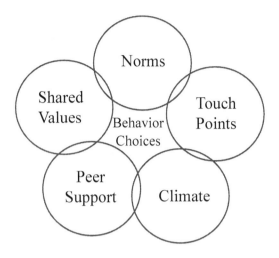

Shared Values

In American culture, the tendency is to think of values on a personal level. It might be said, for example, that a particular person values honesty and hard work. However, groups and organizations also adopt values. Sometimes they are referred to as priorities. The Dell and Intel corporate cultures, for example, value speed of innovation. Southwest Airlines is renowned for a culture that values humor and fun. Most successful companies have cultures that value profitability, customer service and innovation, or some variation on those themes. In a wellness culture, employee well-being makes the top tier of cultural values. The organizational culture embraces the idea that healthy people are an essential piece of the overall corporate strategy. Employees throughout the organization are likely to report that wellness is considered important in their work unit and throughout other parts of the organization.

Norms

Cultural norms are social expectations for behavior and beliefs. Norms are sometimes referred to as "the way we do things around here." Norms tend to form a "cultural unconscious" in that people no longer think of their actions as being influenced by norms. The norm becomes apparent only when it is changing or when someone violates the norm. If you are feeling brave, test a stress management norm at work. During your break sit on the floor with your legs crossed and your eyes closed. Such a healthy practice is likely to result in "push-back" from coworkers. No law has been broken, but norms have their own enforcement mechanisms. Norms are reinforced by the formal and informal mechanisms called cultural touch points we discussed in Chapter 4.

Cultures vary in the strength of their norms. The culture may send clear signals about whether a behavior is a norm. For example, there is a strong norm to wear cloths in most workplaces. Other behaviors such as whether people car pool to work are likely to be weak. The culture is not sending strong signals. Hopefully, as environmental awareness grows, sharing a ride to work will become a stronger norm. A weak culture, one characterized by what we call "anomie," lacks norms for collaboration. Anomie often leaves people feeling overwhelmed and confused. Anomie makes it difficult to function and work productively with others.

A wellness culture supports individual choice and features some norms that make it easier for people to maintain healthy lifestyles. For example, in the area of healthy eating, it would be a norm for the company to serve delicious and nutritious snacks that are low in salt, fat and sugar. In a healthy culture, it would be the norm for people to use their breaks for physical activity, healthy eating, stress management and friendship. Smoking would not be the only acceptable excuse for a break.

Touch Points

Cultural touch points are the mechanisms for maintaining and establishing norms. Ten primary and overlapping touch points shape the culture: (1) rewards and recognition, (2) confrontation,

(3) relationships, (4) modeling, (5) recruitment and selection, (6) orientation, (7) training, (8) communication, (9) rites, rituals and symbols, and (10) resource commitment. The "Aligning Cultural Touch Points" chapter examines these 10 primary touch points and how they can be used to support wellness. They must be understood and adjusted to sustain desired culture change. Touch points include formal policies, procedures and programs as well as informal and unwritten influences. The formal policy of a 40-hour workweek and a daily lunch break, for example, can be overpowered by rewards and praise for going the extra mile.

Peer Support

Peer support is assistance given by friends, housemates, family, coworkers and supervisors. This includes emotional support such as good listening, expressions of enthusiasm and empathy. Peer support also includes instrumental assistance such as offering child care, providing needed equipment and covering for work responsibilities. Teamwork is a synonym for peer support in the workplace. In American culture, peer support is often looked at with suspicion. People who are able to achieve things on their own are seen as more noble. Wellness programs address this cultural attitude by helping people realize that lasting change is more likely when strong individual initiative is combined with effective peer support.

Climate

Three cultural climate factors—a sense of community, a shared vision and a positive outlook—have been found to play important roles in making individual and organizational growth possible. A sense of community is present when people feel as if they belong, care for one another in times of need and get to know one another. A shared vision is present when people are inspired by what they are doing together and feel that they operate from a base of common values. A positive outlook is seen when people fully recognize their individual and collective strengths. People with a positive outlook tend to view their work in terms of challenges and opportunities rather than problems and obstacles. The three climate factors represent the intersection between organizational development and individual wellness. Where the climate factors are noticeably absent, people are so distracted by distrust, anger and negativity that they cannot focus on their own well-being. In an unhealthy climate, organizational goals for innovation, teamwork and service fail to get the follow-through and commitment necessary for success. As an employee working in a negative climate might put it, "why bother?"

Culture Questions

The cultural dimensions were introduced in the opening chapter, "A Call to Wellness Leadership." Together, the five dimensions determine the influence of the culture. As you design your wellness dashboard, the following questions and strategies will be useful in examining the impact of your work subculture.

1. **Has desired wellness behavior become "the way we do things around here?"** Employees can be asked about their level of agreement that wellness norms have been established. A survey such as the Lifegain Health Culture Audit (discussed in the next section) can ask employees about their perceptions of expected behavior. Another measurement strategy is to have a new employee report on his or her early impressions of the workplace. New employees tend to be more aware of how they must adapt to the written and unwritten rules. A third strategy is to ask those with healthy practices to describe any cultural push-back. A similar approach can be used with employees who have unhealthy practices. These employees can be asked about the extent to which their unhealthy behavior is being supported or resisted. From this information, you can determine whether pockets of employees or subcultures have stronger wellness norms. You can also learn if some groups have yet to achieve strong wellness norms.

2. **Has wellness behavior become a top-tier priority within your work group?** You can ask employees about their level of agreement that the wellness goals are broadly shared. In addition to this question, you can ask about the priorities of your work group to determine if wellness has made the list. Observe the communication, budget and decision-making process. Is wellness a part of the discussion of work group and organizational priorities? Your goals are to ensure that wellness is a part of the discussion and to gain employee agreement that wellness behavior is worthy of attention and commitment.

3. **Do peers effectively support wellness behavior goals?** You can ask employees if their coworkers, housemates, family and friends support wellness behavior. Ask employees about their recent lifestyle change attempts. What peer support was available? Who could have been more supportive? How might peers have helped? Do employees pair up or team up to make changes, or must they pursue wellness alone? Your goal is to have social networks support desired behavior by providing emotional and physical assistance.

4. **Do cultural touch points support wellness behavior goals?** Here you are interested in both employee perceptions and formal policies. For example, employees have opinions about whether they are being rewarded and recognized for healthy lifestyle choices. They will also be able to express their views on what can be done to better reward and recognize positive practices. You can use this information to adjust formal policies and to address informal influences. This same approach can be used with all 10 touch points examined in the previous chapter. Your goal is have touch points work to reinforce desired behavior.

5. **Does the overall work climate support constructive change?** It is difficult for people to focus on personal change in hostile environments. Social discord will also make it difficult for your group to implement a wellness program. You can ask employees to rate the sense of community, shared vision and positive outlook in their work group. Your goal is to maintain and strengthen these three work climate factors. A Work Climate Survey and a more complete discussion of how to achieve a healthy work climate is available at www.healthyworkclimate.com.

Measuring Culture with the Lifegain Health Culture Audit

The *Lifegain Health Culture Audit* measures culture as it applies to wellness. The survey is tailored to norm goals and frequently incorporates health behavior, program interest and program evaluation questions. Generic *Lifegain Health Culture Audit* questions used in a short-form version of the anonymous survey follow.

Lifegain Health Culture Audit

Please rate your level of agreement with the following statements on the 5-point scale: (5) strongly agree, (4) agree, (3) undecided/don't know, (2) disagree, and (1) strongly disagree.

5 4 3 2 1	Living a healthy lifestyle is highly valued in my work unit.
5 4 3 2 1	My immediate supervisor models a healthy lifestyle.
5 4 3 2 1	My workplace demonstrates its commitment to supporting healthy lifestyles through its use of resources such as time, space and money.
5 4 3 2 1	People in my work unit are taught skills needed to achieve a healthy lifestyle.
5 4 3 2 1	New employees at my work unit are made aware of the organization's support for healthy lifestyles.

Lifegain Health Culture Audit Continued

Please rate your level of agreement with the following statements on the 5-point scale: (5) strongly agree, (4) agree, (3) undecided/ don't know, (2) disagree, and (1) strongly disagree.

5 4 3 2 1	In my work unit, people are rewarded and recognized for efforts to live a healthy lifestyle.
5 4 3 2 1	In my work unit, participation in healthy activities is a primary way to renew friendships and to meet new people.
5 4 3 2 1	In my work unit, unhealthy behaviors such as smoking and excess drinking are discouraged.
5 4 3 2 1	My work unit has a sense of community (for example, people really get to know one another, feel as if they belong and care for one another in times of need).
5 4 3 2 1	My work unit has a shared vision (for example, people feel that the organization's conduct is consistent with their personal values and people are clear about how they fit in with the big picture).
5 4 3 2 1	My work unit has a positive outlook (for example, people enjoy their work, celebrate accomplishments, adopt a "we can do it" attitude and bring out the best in each other).
5 4 3 2 1	My immediate supervisor supports employees' efforts to adopt healthier lifestyle practices.
5 4 3 2 1	My immediate coworkers support one another's efforts to adopt healthier lifestyle practices.
5 4 3 2 1	My friends, family members and/or housemates support one another's efforts to adopt healthier lifestyle practices.

Lifegain Health Culture Audit Continued

Please rate your level of agreement with the following statements on the 5-point scale: (5) strongly agree, (4) agree, (3) undecided/don't know, (2) disagree, and (1) strongly disagree.

In my immediate work unit, it is a norm (expected) for people to...	
5 4 3 2 1	Be physically active (such as taking a brisk walk for 30 minutes most days).
5 4 3 2 1	Get adequate sleep (seven-plus hours).
5 4 3 2 1	Achieve a balance between work, rest and play.
5 4 3 2 1	Eat amounts of food that maintain a healthy weight.
5 4 3 2 1	Eat foods that are low in fat and refined sugar and high in whole grains, fruits and vegetables.
5 4 3 2 1	Drink alcohol moderately, if at all.
5 4 3 2 1	Use car safety belts.
5 4 3 2 1	Follow safety precautions at work (including practicing good lifting techniques and organizing the work environment to avoid injury).
5 4 3 2 1	Not smoke.
5 4 3 2 1	Not come to work sick.
5 4 3 2 1	Stay current on medical screenings.

The *Lifegain Health Culture Audit* assesses all five cultural dimensions. The first question asks about shared values. Questions 2 to 8 examine cultural touch points. Questions 9 to 11 assess the work climate. Questions 12 to 14 ask about peer support. Question 14 to 25 questions ask about existing cultural norms. For all items, higher scores indicate stronger support for healthy practices. An average score of 3 on any of the norm questions indicates that the culture is not sending clear signals for or against a healthy lifestyle practice. A score below 3 indicates that the norm supports an unhealthy practice.

Learning Assignment

Developing Cultural Measures

Your wellness dashboard should show that the culture supports healthy lifestyles.

How will you measure wellness norms?

How will you assess shared wellness values to determine if wellness is a top-tier priority?

How will you assess the quantity and quality of peer support for healthy lifestyles?

How will you assess the 10 cultural touch points?

How will you assess the work climate?

Adopting a Principled Approach to Data Gathering

You need to know that your wellness efforts are working. Regular and accurate feedback helps you adjust failed strategies. It keeps you focused on what is working. And a sound information base will justify continued commitment by you, your work group and your organization. The following principles should guide your efforts.

- **Link decisions to information.** Generate a steady flow of information and be sure to follow up on the findings. This will take much of the guesswork out of your efforts.

- **Incorporate both qualitative and quantitative assessment.** Quantitative data are measurable through counting. Quantitative data allows you to summarize the impact of your efforts. Qualitative data is descriptive information. The qualitative data includes success stories that will inspire.

- **Limit your data gathering so that you do not waste time and money.** Too much of the wrong information will distract rather than inform. Asking for unneeded information is a turnoff.

- **Respect privacy and the law.** People don't want to feel watched and, as discussed in Appendix B, there are legal safeguards that prevent employers from misusing health information. Your organization doesn't need, nor should it have, personal health information that is not voluntarily shared with full and explicit consent.

Making Feedback Positive

Most wellness concerns begin with the negative. For example, someone might express concern about her weight. An employer might be distressed about the rising cost of medical care. Wellness is about moving these negatives in positive directions. When you help your employees celebrate success, it does not mean you are overlooking remaining problems. It means that you are deemphasizing individual fault and blame. Your challenge is to refocus attention on constructive change. Determine what can be done both individually and collectively to proactively achieve better wellness outcomes.

Build on individual and group strengths. Focus on personal health assets and the capacity to support lifestyle change. Both feedback and planning should be organized around strengths rather than weaknesses. Strengths help individuals and organizations move forward. To see how this works, take a concern and come up with all the positive resources that may be brought to bear on that concern. This contrasts with how most people handle change. Your positive approach will feel fresh and constructive.

People respond to praise and encouragement. Try not to let successes go unacknowledged. Ask for permission to publicly acknowledge your employees' efforts. Unheralded success does more than undercut good cheer. It signals a missed opportunity to reinforce desired practices.

Workplaces and individuals thrive within a culture of optimism and enthusiasm. Wellness programs can foster a positive outlook by emphasizing productive potential and teaching people how to overcome obstacles.

Many Americans have a "can do" attitude. This is a helpful cultural trait when it comes to attempting lifestyle improvements. Positive personal change is both expected and celebrated.

American individualism sends mixed signals about whether it is OK to discuss personal changes. Men, for example, are sometimes considered more masculine if they achieve goals through personal will and without assistance. Although the Internet seems to be creating more public forums for our personal affairs, many people refrain from such public discussions of personal goals. For many people, daily practices are considered private endeavors, and sharing progress is called bragging. An undesirable side effect of the go it alone approach is that no one even knows when benchmarks are set, let alone achieved. Advocates of the quiet approach go on to praise the value of self-achievement and self-responsibility as if help from others somehow taints successful behavior change and downgrades the achievement. The ability to say "I did it entirely on my own" gives one special bragging rights. Often when someone does it on his own, it is also a sign of a disconnected society and a strong indication that the changes will be short-lived. We want and need to celebrate together.

Celebrating All Along the Way

Seek opportunities to celebrate wellness—there are many to be found. They go well beyond the typical approach of celebrating only when the ultimate goal is achieved. Consider the possibilities for celebrating success when:

- A survey or self-assessment reveals that your employees have many great wellness strengths.

- An employee sets a wellness goal.

- Someone finds a good wellness role model.

- Some barrier to wellness is eliminated.

- Someone finds people and places that will support her wellness goal.

- Someone develops strategies for limiting contact with unsupportive environments.

- Someone gets back on track after a relapse.

- It is the anniversary of a significant wellness achievement.

Learning Assignment

Maintaining a Positive Approach

Breaking with negativity requires some effort. With a little creativity and persistence, your wellness program can be a positive force for change.

How will you use positive language and framing to express wellness initiatives and goals?

How will you take full advantage of individual and group strengths when approaching needed changes?

How will you make sure that progress is celebrated?

Appreciating Intrinsic and Extrinsic Rewards

Good celebrations often include rewards. Such rewards come in two forms: **intrinsic** and **extrinsic**. Although this subject came up in "Aligning Cultural Touch Points," it has particular relevance to your efforts to monitor and celebrate success. An intrinsic reward is a benefit that directly results from behavior change, for example, feeling more energetic after becoming fit. An extrinsic reward is a benefit from an outside source. The 30-day sobriety chip of Alcoholics Anonymous would be an example of an extrinsic reward.

Most wellness goals result in multiple intrinsic rewards. A breast cancer survivor, for example, has the obvious intrinsic rewards of a longer life and freedom from cancer signs and symptoms. Another reward is new knowledge and skills that can be used for managing other great personal threats and challenges. The experience may also have resulted in self-discovery and an opportunity to establish new personal priorities. These would all be intrinsic rewards.

You can help your employees explore the intrinsic rewards likely to result from achieving their wellness goals. Ask them about the intrinsic benefits. Achieving wellness goals lowers the probability of getting sick and reduces recovery time when one does get sick. In addition, many wellness-related behavior changes improve job performance and mood. Sometimes our wellness achievements directly benefit those we love. Stopping smoking, for example, improves health outcomes for our children.

Some benefits are surprising. Did you know that quitting smoking improves sexual performance? (In most workplaces it is probably better that you not bring this up. Let your employees discover the quirkier intrinsic rewards.) A lot of scientific information is available on the various health consequences of unhealthy and healthy behaviors. You can review this information to uncover some wonderful rewards that result from healthier lifestyles.

Extrinsic rewards are the way peers, groups and society reinforce wellness. For example, you could reward wellness achievements with praise, a card or some other form of acknowledgment. Similar informal rewards are available from other peers, such as family, friends and housemates. For example, a man who has lowered his cholesterol might comment that one great reward was the look on his wife's face when the results came back.

Organizations and society also have rewards for wellness activities, such as incentives for completing company health risk appraisals. Good health could lead to job promotions, since advancement is often linked to personal productivity and we tend to be a lot less productive when we are sick. There are also rewards associated with competitions. Examples include T-shirts and medals people get for competing in fitness events.

Sometimes extrinsic rewards for wellness are criticized because they are considered a distraction from intrinsic rewards. Other criticisms concern how external rewards are often temporary and are not controlled by the person making the change. It does at first appear odd to "pay" someone for doing something that offers great intrinsic health benefits. However, in most cases it is best to mix intrinsic and extrinsic rewards. For example, stopping smoking is a great accomplishment with direct intrinsic health benefits for those who quit. However, external rewards, such as lowered health insurance deductibles for nonsmokers, do not undermine the intrinsic rewards. External rewards just make the behavior change even more rewarding and are likely to get the attention of those who have yet to pay attention to the intrinsic rewards.

We can help people tune in to the intrinsic health and self-esteem rewards and make sure that they get all the external perks, pay and praise available for their achievements.

Refining the Reward Systems

As can be seen with the list of reasons to celebrate and with the variety of intrinsic and extrinsic rewards available, there are many ways to make celebrations meaningful and appropriate. The following questions can help you tailor celebrations to best suit your people's needs.

- **What is the best way to handle privacy?** As a general rule, public disclosure and commitment work in favor of successful behavior change. It is a lot harder to give up or go back once you have declared your intentions and progress. However, your employees may not want particular people to know about any changes under way. Who should and should not know? How can we celebrate and yet maintain desired confidentiality?

- **How can we make rewards compatible with wellness?** In American culture, many common rewards are inconsistent with a wellness message. For example, a piece of cake is not an appropriate extrinsic reward for successful weight management. Exotic fruits and vegetables make a good alternative. A new outfit could be a more fitting reward. We must often be creative and willing to break with tradition to create a wellness reward system.

- **Are there savings that can be applied toward financing a grand prize?** When I (Judd) stopped drinking diet soda and fancy coffees, I put the money into a travel fund. In the course of a couple of years, these savings made it possible for me to take my grandmother on a cruise to Alaska. See if your employees' achievements offer some savings or another financial benefit. Avoiding illness adds to productivity and reduces costs. Can some or all of this money be redirected toward a fitting reward?

- **What are the favorite ways to celebrate?** We all have our preferences—our favorite way to relax, our favorite healthy foods, our favorite way to exercise, our favorite places. Rewards should be tailored to personal taste. What is the nicest thing anyone ever said to your employee? Maybe the tone and spirit of that comment can be mirrored in how wellness achievements are celebrated. For example, I found it particularly satisfying when my father talked to me in private about how proud he was of my professional achievements. I favor similar private acknowledgments of current wellness achievements. Some people find monetary rewards most meaningful. If this is the case, a good celebration includes cash or a check.

- **Are there special celebrants?** Perhaps certain esteemed friends, family members or coworkers would offer particularly meaningful rewards—intrinsic or otherwise. Expressions of delight from a spouse, an "attagirl" from the boss, or praise from Mom and Dad may carry special weight.

Monitoring and Celebrating Success Checklist

☐ Develop your performance, programmatic and cultural measures. How will you assess behavior change? How will you assess the benefits to the organization? How will you know that people are participating in the program? How will you get feedback on the quality and appropriateness of wellness programs? How will you know that changes to policies and procedures have been implemented successfully? How will you know that the culture now supports wellness?

☐ Plan your strategies for celebrating success. How will you honor individual contributions to the initiative? How will you tailor rewards to individual needs? How will you call attention to intrinsic and extrinsic rewards? How will you celebrate the achievements of your work group?

Leadership Stories

◆ Jose was proud of his team's progress. The results from the annual culture survey were in. Sixty-three percent of employees agreed or strongly agreed that they were being rewarded and recognized for healthier lifestyles. Survey feedback also indicated that training, resource commitment, leadership modeling and orientation were now working toward wellness. The largest need was seen in peer support. A peer mentoring initiative was being planned to address this need.

◆ It took some doing, but the results at Zimbardo and Stone, LLC have been outstanding. The law firm had focused on five behaviors: not smoking, healthy eating, regular physical activity, work/life balance and moderate drinking. Three years ago, just 23 percent of employees had reported attaining all five health assets. Now the results were 53 percent. An amazing 73 percent reported four of the five assets.

◆ Janet was thrilled that her department had achieved yet another well workplace award. There was a lot of excitement about the annual awards ceremony. The new university president would be there. She wondered how her team would spend the money. Last year they all went to the Spa at Topnotch.

◆ Mike's work group was really on track. He wanted his people to get a sense of what was available through the wellness program. All but 10 of his employees had met with a wellness coach at least once for an initial assessment and consult. He would send a reminder to the holdouts. He was also able to recruit two members of his team for the company wellness committee. The needs of his work group would be heard.

◆ Alice was pleased about Jan's new walking routine. Jan had struggled with her weight and now was making real progress. Alice asked Jan how she would be celebrating. Jan smiled as she said, "Don't tell anyone, but I'm getting a whole new wardrobe."

Chapter 6: Full Engagement

Great wellness initiatives engage the vast majority of employees by:

- Creating conditions that achieve immediate goals and lasting results.

- Responding to changing organizational needs and business conditions.

- Utilizing best practices and available research.

- Making efficient use of time, space, money and other resources.

- Serving the whole person and diverse individual lifestyle change needs.

- Operating in a way that is thoughtful, inspirational and fun.

There are many moving parts in a great wellness program. As can be inferred from the Lifestyle Assessment Inventory presented in the chapter "Serving as an Effective Role Model," there are many hundreds of lifestyle change combinations. The complexity doesn't end with the fact that wellness goals are unique. Organizations are complex systems with unique traditions, subcultures and challenges. This complexity and diversity ensure that there is no one perfect wellness program model. A great wellness program requires knowledgeable wellness champions, collaboration, adaptation and a systematic approach. Such an organized approach reduces the likelihood of confusion and maximizes opportunities for cooperation.

Most often the creation of a wellness program also involves developing wellness committees and hiring wellness professionals. These committees and professionals have responsibilities that go beyond the core leadership skills described in the preceding *Wellness Leadership* chapters.

This chapter, "Full Engagement," offers a conceptual map for wellness program design and implementation. You may or may not be responsible for organizing a wellness program, but some basic understanding of the mechanics will help you determine your wellness leadership role and how you might support your organization's wellness initiative.

The Role of Wellness Committees

A typical wellness committee is a small group (fewer than 15 members) of wellness champions who coordinate wellness promotion. In a very large organization, each setting may have a wellness committee. In a very small organization, the responsibilities may be assigned to a handful of individuals or the person responsible for human resources functions. The primary responsibilities of wellness committees are to:

- Develop broad support for the wellness initiative and foster participation by seeing to it that the wellness program serves most or all employee groups. The committee must articulate a compelling and inclusive vision for the wellness initiative. It should ensure that employees are kept informed about the wellness program and that all employees can benefit from the program.

- Work with wellness professionals to develop an annual

plan and budget for the wellness program. This includes helping to determine annual performance, programmatic and cultural goals (see "Monitoring and Celebrating Success"). Responsibilities also include assisting with the selection and management of professional wellness services and the purchase of wellness resources.

- Develop a communication plan whereby employees at all levels are made aware of the program and are encouraged to adopt healthier lifestyles.

- Incorporate best practices and promising wellness ideas into the wellness initiative. Committee members seek out the best approaches and information by looking both internally and at what is being done in other organizations. The committee should adapt and disseminate these innovative ideas and practices.

- Develop methods for assessing the wellness program and for celebrating progress that has been achieved. The wellness committee is responsible for making sure that people get the feedback they need to fully appreciate the results and improve their efforts.

Composition

The wellness committee should be diverse in composition so that the program can gain input from throughout the organization. It should include representatives from a cross-section of employee groups as well as human resources professionals responsible for setting other organizational policies and procedures. The committee should have union representation (when available) and employees from all shifts and work locations. If there are distinct professional groups, then each group should be represented. The committee structure may include wellness professionals, but it is also appropriate to include these professionals as non-voting members.

Members of the wellness committee should have a reputation for good leadership skills and should have earned the respect of their peers and organizational leaders. All committee members should be wellness enthusiasts. Committee members can be nominated by employee groups and by organizational leaders.

It is recommended that the term of membership be one year. This provides for rotating membership. Having terms makes membership transitions less awkward. However, committee members could be invited to continue for multiple terms. The committee should have co-chairs and someone responsible for administrative functions (e.g., scheduling, recording minutes and managing communication). Subcommittees are often established. Standing subcommittees could, for example, be established to handle the budget, communication, personnel and special projects.

Although there are no hard rules about the size of a wellness committee, it is generally agreed that committees over a certain size become unwieldy. A dozen members is a good target. In a large or widespread organization, multiple committees are recommended. A committee with more than 15 members will find it difficult to get input from the entire group. A committee with just a handful of members may find itself overwhelmed.

Logistics

It is recommended that wellness committees meet at least monthly. A two-hour time slot should be scheduled for meetings. The location of the meetings should allow for privacy and a minimum of interruptions. An agenda should be prepared in advance, and committee members should be given an opportunity to add to this agenda. A typical agenda includes time for catching up on personal news, a review of the minutes from the previous meeting, subcommittee reports, reports on special projects and discussion of new ideas. The co-chairs should take responsibility for facilitating meetings.

Training

Wellness committee members should be trained in how to: (1) develop and share the wellness program vision, (2) serve as effective role models, (3) align cultural touch points, and (4) monitor and celebrate success. *Wellness Leadership* could be used for teaching these basic leadership skills. It is recommended that a new wellness committee begin its work by answering the questions presented as assignments in each *Wellness Leadership* chapter. Answering the questions will help familiarize committee members with key wellness ideas and give each member an opportunity to weigh in on his wellness program preferences. Feedback for answers to the *Wellness Leadership* questions is available by registering for the online Wellness Leadership Training (www.leadwellness.com).

Established wellness committees should have a strategy for orienting and training new members.

- A packet of information about the wellness program should be made available to new members; it should include the minutes of past wellness committee meetings.

- New members could be encouraged to read *Wellness Leadership* and to learn how key leadership questions are being addressed.

- A committee member could serve as a mentor to the new member and be available for discussions. The new member should be encouraged to get acquainted with each committee member.

It is recommended that ongoing training be made available to all committee members. These training experiences will help keep programming ideas fresh. They will also bring in new perspectives and challenge prevailing wisdom. For example, committee members could attend local and national conferences and then report to the committee on what they learned. The National Wellness

Conference (www.nationalwellness.org) held each July in Stevens Point, Wisconsin would be a good choice for annual enrichment and renewal. The Art of Health Promotion Conference sponsored by the *American Journal of Health Promotion* is another good option (www.healthpromotionjournal.com).

Training should include lessons about best practices. Textbooks, journal articles and lectures frequently offer best practices data. Although the best practices recommendations tend to be fairly unspecific and broad, they are likely to be great food for thought and to increase confidence. For example, it is common for best practices studies to report that a supportive environment and leadership support are keys to success. This message would be encouraging for those of us interested in wellness leadership and cultural touch points.

You can deepen your appreciation of best practices by visiting those organizations that have been identified as having outstanding wellness programs. Reaching out to other organizations is likely to lead to collaboration and a level of learning that goes beyond what is available in the literature.

Hopefully, you will have an opportunity to return the favor by assisting another organization looking for guidance. A review of your own best practices is likely to strengthen your wellness program. You are likely to gain clarity about your efforts, and helping others builds self-esteem. Your support also helps to build the wellness movement.

Learning Assignment

Forming and Maintaining a Wellness Committee

Wellness committees play important roles in many wellness programs. Consider some of the ways your committee can help ensure the effectiveness of a wellness committee.

What is the composition of the wellness committee? Is it made up of enthusiastic, capable and diverse leaders?

Does the wellness committee feel sufficiently clear about its role? Does the committee feel empowered?

How does the wellness committee deepen its knowledge and skills? Is training available? Can best practices lead the way?

The Role of Wellness Professionals

Wellness professionals create a wide range of services and resources, including testing, newsletters, health information Web sites, support group facilitation, training and wellness coaching. Many larger organizations hire their own internal wellness professional teams to manage and deliver wellness programming. It is also common for organizations to utilize the professional services of health insurers and wellness companies.

Wellness professionals often play a lead role in program design and delivery. For example, they develop ways to communicate the wellness program vision, including information about the benefits of the wellness program and information about how employees can participate. These professionals should actively develop strategies for addressing cultural touch points. They should offer policy recommendations, programs and other services to address the touch points.

Wellness professionals play a further role in offering wellness counseling or coaching. They meet employees in person, over the phone and online to discuss wellness goals. These coaching or counseling services help employees set goals, gather key health information and stay on track.

Wellness professionals, wellness departments and external wellness providers usually collect workers' health information. For legal reasons and to maintain confidentiality, this data needs to be kept private. For a more complete explanation of the legal issues, see Appendix B. The wellness professional can and should provide aggregate data that does not disclose individual employee responses. In addition, the wellness professional can organize the data, conduct statistical comparisons and compare findings over time or against benchmarks. This information can help you track your work group's progress.

Learning Assignment

Utilizing Wellness Professionals

Your work group could benefit from professional support. Consider which functions these wellness professionals should provide your group.

What professional wellness services are already available to your employees through your employer, through insurance companies and through community resources?

What additional professional services would be useful in helping your employees achieve their wellness goals?

What could be done to make better use of current professional resources?

Adopting a Systematic Approach

The wellness program is organized to bring about a well workplace culture. Just as the word culture originates from the concept of cultivation, bringing about culture change is similar to good farming practices. A farmer knows to examine the soil. He knows to prepare the soil for planting. He knows the best time and way to plant the seed, and he knows how to nurture the growing crop. Such a capable farmer also knows when to harvest and how to leave the soil fertile. The following graphic and descriptions show these same phases as they apply to cultivating a well workplace culture.

The Normative Systems Culture Change Process

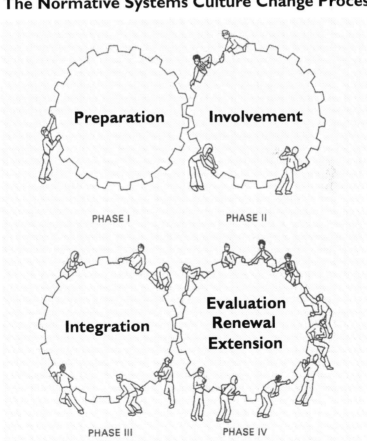

Preparation

Involvement

PHASE I

PHASE II

Integration

Evaluation Renewal Extension

PHASE III

PHASE IV

Phase I: Preparation

What will be the vision of success? What values, norms and behaviors will be primary? What wellness benefits will be emphasized?

What will be the baseline measures?

Who will be the champions and how will leadership be developed?

What will be done to align cultural touch points?

What will be the pace and timing of the culture change effort?

Phase II: Involvement

How will the wellness initiative be described?

How will wellness champions and managers express their enthusiasm for the effort?

How will employees be invited to participate?

What will be said about how cultural touch points will be aligned?

Phase III: Integration

What changes in organizational policies and procedures will go into effect?

How will peer support be mobilized?

What professional wellness services will be available?

What will be done with community resources?

Phase IV: Evaluation, Renewal and Extension

How will individual and collective change be assessed?

What will be the feedback mechanism?

How will progress be celebrated?

What will be done to build on what has been achieved?

As seen in the questions that are addressed in each phase, managing wellness is an ongoing, evolving process. There are many pieces to an effective program, and an overarching change process offers a framework for coordinating these efforts. It is recommended that all phases be carried out on an annual cycle. Each cycle allows for a change in wellness goals and strategies. Such a framework makes it easier to explain how the program works and how people can get involved.

Learning Assignment

Developing a Systematic Approach

A systematic and businesslike approach increases the likelihood of achieving a well workplace culture. You can help see to it that the wellness initiative is well organized and systematic.

How is the wellness program organized?

What are the phases and what is the timeline for each phase of the wellness initiative?

Do employees know about the phases and how they can participate in each phase?

Developing Managers and Employees

A good wellness program has a constructive role for everyone. You can assist in developing roles for managers and other employees. A discussion of two approaches follows.

Wellness Leadership Training

The central goal of *Wellness Leadership* is to explain how managers at every level can better support a well workplace. The book is useful for managers seeking to play a constructive role. These skills could be reinforced with online and classroom training that develops skills for: (1) sharing the wellness vision, (2) serving as a role model, (3) aligning cultural touch points, and (4) monitoring and celebrating success. The Wellness Leadership Training includes testimonials and other resource materials. Information about offering Wellness Leadership Training is available at www.leadwellness.com.

Wellness Mentor Program

Employees can play a constructive role by engaging in effective peer support for lifestyle change. Peer support is important to a well workplace culture, and peer support skills have the advantage of extending wellness program benefits to employees' households. *Healthy Habits, Helpful Friends* is about offering such support. In addition, a worksite Wellness Mentor Program can be offered whereby employees are trained to offer peer support. The training is available in both classroom and online formats. A wellness mentor program often includes mechanisms for matching up peers for mentoring. This is a good follow-up option for employee health surveys. Typically, employees are matched for mutual support. Information about creating a Wellness Mentor Program is available at www.healthyculture.com.

> ### Learning Assignment
>
> ### Developing Supportive Wellness Roles
>
> Wellness enthusiasts need a constructive way to promote wellness. You can help give all employees opportunities to get involved.
>
> How will executives, managers and supervisors develop their capacity to support wellness?
>
> What role can those employees without supervisory responsibilities play in supporting wellness?

Maintaining Open Communication

Those responsible for coordinating and delivering wellness programs need to maintain good relationships with managers and other organizational leaders to do their jobs effectively. Similarly, managers should keep abreast of wellness program developments so that their employees get the full benefit of the wellness program. The following suggestions will help maximize this collaborative relationship:

- Establish a communication mechanism for keeping current on wellness program activities. Managers need to know what is available and how their employees can enroll in these activities.

- Each *Wellness Leadership* chapter poses questions and assignments that are useful in developing the leadership role of managers. Managers should consult wellness program coordinators (such as wellness professionals and committee members) about answers to these questions. This will result in better coordination, constructive insights and a stronger shared vision of the program.

- When information is collected from your employees, managers should get aggregate feedback about their work group. Managers should share these findings with employees. This completes the feedback loop and lets your employees know that their opinions count.

- Those responsible for coordinating and delivering wellness programs can share success stories and lists of role models. Sharing this information enhances enthusiasm and increases acceptance of the wellness program.

- Managers should give those responsible for coordinating and delivering wellness programs constructive feedback about the wellness program. Proximity to day-to-day activities is likely to give managers an important and useful perspective on how wellness programs can be improved.

- Managers should not expect those responsible for coordinating and delivering wellness programs to single-handedly create a wellness culture. A wellness culture is a shared responsibility. Employees at all levels need to be proactive in fostering a wellness culture.

Learning Assignment

Wellness Program Communication

Those responsible for coordinating the wellness program need to coordinate and communicate with managers at all levels.

What will be done to keep mangers abreast of what is happening in the wellness program?

What will be done to create a good feedback loop between managers and those responsible for organizing the wellness program?

Full Engagement Checklist

☐ Describe your efforts to form and mobilize wellness committees. Who should serve on the wellness committee and why?
How will the right people be recruited to serve? What training will be available for the wellness committee? How will the
committee get resources needed to make the program successful?

☐ Describe your use of wellness professionals. Who will help
evaluate your wellness program? Who will deliver counseling
and other individualized behavior change services? How will
your program interact with community wellness resources
and insurers such as health clubs, municipal parks and rec-
reation departments and other local wellness vendors? How
will insurance and medical providers support the wellness
program? Who will manage and coordinate these professional
resources?

☐ Describe your efforts to adopt a systematic approach. What
will be done for analysis, objective setting and leadership
development? How will employees be first engaged in the
wellness effort? What will be done to create environmental
conditions that support employees' efforts? How will the program be evaluated and celebrated? When will the next round
of culture change be planned? What is the timeline for the
full cycle of the wellness initiative?

☐ Describe how you will empower wellness champions to get
involved in the wellness program. What will be done to get
managers involved and trained? What will be done to give
other employees a constructive role?

Leadership Stories

◆ Laura had been wellness director for more than 20 years. At this point, most of the program ran like clockwork. The annual report came out in January. It included a summary of the previous year's efforts as well as the plan for the coming year. The program remained nimble and highly adaptable to the changing needs of the workforce. This year's emphasis was on physical activity. Achieving national objectives for regular physical activity had taken some doing. Next year's goals for reducing fatigue were equally daunting. The broader culture was way off. It was not a norm to get adequate sleep, and the night-shift workers were especially challenged.

◆ Spike's wellness committee never quite clicked. Committee members began with a great deal of enthusiasm. They never developed a mission or strategic plan, however. There were a lot of program ideas, but nobody really had any training. The committee budget amounted to less than $5 per employee. The wellness program looked like a laundry list of inexpensive and poorly implemented activities. It was easy to see that the committee would soon exhaust itself without having achieved any lasting results.

◆ The High on Wellness Corporation offered a turnkey service. All employees were invited to take an online health survey. Reports with lifestyle recommendations were generated. A master report was sent to the human resource department with ROI forecasts. The high-risk employees were called by a wellness coach, and other employees were sent e-mails with links to online health information. Unfortunately, few employees participated and results were short-lived. It looked good on paper and it was affordable. However, nothing was done to change the work environment, and employees were not engaged in supporting the program.

◆ Jennet liked that she was not the only one fired up about wellness. She had identified a number of wellness champions and they all had constructive roles. Some served on the worksite wellness committee. Others had received Wellness Leadership Training or had become wellness mentors. Leadership support was particularly helpful in getting employee participation and in implementing new wellness policies. The mentors were spreading wellness throughout the organization. In addition, peer support had become a great mechanism for raising lifestyle change success rates.

Glossary

Barriers to Change – Successful behavior change frequently requires resources such as time, equipment, mental focus and the cooperation of others. Lack of needed resources makes it difficult to modify behavior and constitutes a barrier to change. You can help your employees cope with, overcome and eliminate barriers to change.

Cultural Climate – A sense of community, a shared vision and a positive outlook are social environmental factors that enhance the capacity of individuals and organizations to grow. A sense of community provides for trust and openness. A shared vision enables people to be inspired by a common direction. A positive outlook makes it possible to use individual and collective strengths in meeting challenges. Together, these factors constitute the cultural climate that is present at work, at home or in the community. Workplace wellness programs work best when they limit exposure to unhealthy climates and increase exposure to healthy ones.

Cultural Norms – The accepted and expected behavior of a culture. Sometimes such behaviors are referred to as "the way we do things around here." People are most likely to be aware of norms when they are new to a culture and are wondering how they are expected to behave. You can help determine whether norms in the workplace support desired healthy behavior. Goals could be set for reducing contact with subcultures that have unsupportive norms. You can also identify groups that have strong norms for desired health behavior. For example, someone seeking to be physically active is likely to benefit from becoming a member of a walking group.

Cultural Touch Points – Subcultures and the broader society influence behavior through broad and overlapping mechanisms called "touch points." The 10 touch points are: (1) rewards and recognition, (2) confrontation, (3) relationships, including teams and friendships, (4) modeling, (5) recruitment and selection, (6) orientation, (7) training, (8) communication, including what is talked about and measured, (9) rites, rituals and symbols, including holidays, events and important stories, and (10) resource commitment, including how time and money are spent. You examine these touch points to determine how workplace influences support or fail to support behavior change goals. Your company's wellness program should work to ensure that it fully supports desired behavior.

Extrinsic Rewards – Peers, groups and society reinforce positive behavior through social recognition, benefits, incentives or other forms of payment. These rewards are known as extrinsic because they are provided by others. Prizes, praise, job promotion and salaries are examples of extrinsic rewards. You can provide praise and other extrinsic rewards for coworkers' progress toward their health behavior change. You may also be helpful in seeking out the extrinsic rewards that may be available for achieving healthy lifestyle goals.

Health and Productivity Management – This program philosophy seeks to integrate all health-related human resources functions including health benefits, disability management, employee assistance and wellness, for the purpose of raising human performance and saving cost. More information about this approach is available from the Institute for Health and Productivity Management (www.ihpm.org).

Intrinsic Rewards – Healthy behaviors offer varied benefits to the changer. An intrinsic reward is a benefit that directly results from behavior change, such as feeling more energetic after becoming more fit. An ex-smoker gets fewer colds, a longer life expectancy, improved athletic performance and a reduced risk of becoming impotent (for men). This is over and above the new freedom and lowered expense of breaking the smoking addiction. You can assist in identifying the many positive rewards that are the direct result of the new health behavior.

Peers – Coworkers, spouses, housemates, friends, neighbors and co-participants in rehabilitation, health or wellness programs have interests and experiences in common. Peers have similar standing and power. Peers are the people in our groups, workplaces and communities whom we view as equals. Our peers can play important roles in helping us achieve personal goals.

Relapse – People often revert to previous, undesired practices when attempting to change unhealthy habits. These setbacks are called "relapses." Workplace wellness programs can help limit relapses by teaching employees strategies for coping with and avoiding difficult situations. When relapse occurs, coworkers can assist one another with getting back on track, limiting self-doubt and guilt, and adjusting change tactics.

Role Model – An employee who has a behavior change goal should know that it's likely that someone has achieved the same goal under very similar circumstances. A person who has achieved such a change could become a role model if she is willing to tell her story. A lot can be learned from such success experiences. They are proof that change is possible and desirable. Role models can explain what worked and what did not work for them. You do not need to be the role model for your employee. You can help find and interview potential role models.

Stages of Behavior Change – Successful behavior change tends to follow this six-step progression. The first stage of behavior change is devoted to developing the reasons for making the change. Stage two involves picking a time for making the change. The third stage involves selecting the strategies for making the change. Stage four is the action stage when behavior begins to change. Stage five is focused on keeping the new behavior going. The final or sixth stage is a time when the new desired behavior is firmly in place and the person is ready to move on to other goals. Your company's wellness program can help to determine where employees are in the change process so that appropriate goals and tasks can be set. You can also celebrate success along the way and use the stages of behavior change to reestablish progress after any relapse.

Wellness – People can consciously choose to live in ways that maximize their health, quality of life and personal performance. Personal wellness is multidimensional and holistic, encompassing mental and physical well-being as well as a person's relationships with others and nature. You can assist your employees in setting personally satisfying wellness goals that are both positive and affirming.

Wellness-related Peer Support – Listening and offering words of encouragement are typical forms of support given by friends, family and coworkers helping others achieve healthy habits. Peer support goes beyond such assistance by strategically focusing on a full range of lifestyle change support, including help with setting goals, eliminating barriers to change, identifying role models, locating supportive environments, working through relapse and celebrating success. Follow-through is another distinctive feature of peers' wellness-related support. They meet regularly to keep behavior change moving forward.

Appendix A: Sample Survey Questions

Sample Health Practices Questions (Yes or No)

1. Do you exercise strenuously (that is, so you breathe heavily and your heart rate goes up for a period lasting at least 20 minutes) at least three times a week?

2. Do you drink alcohol? (If your answer is NO, skip to question 6)

3. Do you feel you should cut down on your drinking?

4. Do people annoy you by criticizing your drinking?

5. From time to time, do you take a drink first thing in the morning to steady your nerves or get rid of a hangover?

6. Do you use nonprescription "recreational" drugs? (If your answer is NO, skip to question 9)

7. Do you feel you should cut down on your drug consumption?

8. Do people annoy you by criticizing your taking of drugs?

9. Do you smoke?

10. Is it difficult for you to balance work, rest and play?

11. Do you feel "blue" a lot of the time?

12. Do you feel like you're making a contribution to the world around you?

13. Do you socialize with close friends, relatives or neighbors at least once a week?

14. Do you eat a low-fat diet?

15. Do you eat a high-fiber diet?

16. Do you consider yourself to be within an ideal weight range (within 10 pounds of a healthy weight)?

17. Do you wear a seat belt at all times when you are in a car?

18. Do you keep current on health screenings and physicals?

19. Do you go to a dentist at least once a year for treatment or a checkup?

Sample Program Interest Questions

1. What three wellness program formats would best meet your needs?

☐ In-person seminars

☐ Health screenings

☐ Support groups

☐ Sports teams and competitions

☐ Organized fitness activities (such as walks, aerobics)

☐ Online information and classes

☐ DVDs and e-books

☐ Written health materials

☐ Hotline

☐ Health library

☐ Other_____

2. What six health subjects are you most interested in?

☐ Smoking cessation

☐ Healthy aging

☐ Back care

☐ Financial health

☐ Beating depression

☐ Losing weight

☐ Cholesterol control

☐ Heart-healthy lifestyle

☐ Exercise/aerobics/fitness

☐ First aid/CPR

☐ Humor in the workplace

☐ Blood pressure control

☐ Women's health

☐ Men's health

☐ Healthy cooking

☐ Stress management

☐ Healthy parenting

☐ Retirement planning

☐ Elder care

☐ Self care (how and when to seek medical care)

☐ Other_____

3. What times could you typically attend a wellness activity? (Check all that apply)

☐ Morning

☐ Lunchtime

☐ Afternoon

☐ Evening

☐ Other_____

4. Would you like wellness programs offered to your partner/spouse/family?

☐ Yes

☐ No

☐ Not applicable

5. Where would be the best location for you to receive lifestyle counseling on the phone?

☐ At work

☐ At home

☐ Not at all

6. Do you have access to the Internet at a location that is suitable for addressing your wellness goals?

☐ Yes

☐ No

☐ Not applicable

7. What are the barriers to your participating in wellness activities at work? (Check all that apply)

☐ Lack of facilities and equipment

☐ Lack of child care

☐ Cost (fees, lost work time)

☐ Distance from home

☐ Transportation

☐ Low comfort with social atmosphere

☐ Not allowed/no support from management

☐ Schedule conflicts

☐ Other_____

Sample Program Evaluation Questions

Please rate your wellness program experience.

Name of wellness activity _____

Dates of activity _____

What is your level of satisfaction on a 5-point scale (5 for totally satisfied and 1 for totally dissatisfied)? _____

Would you recommend the activity to others?

What were the primary strengths of the activity? _____

How might you improve the activity? _____

Appendix B: Legal Considerations

A number of state and federal laws protect employees against violation of their personal privacy, personal liberties and discrimination. Fortunately, a wellness philosophy that promotes personal choice and supportive environments is highly compatible with the spirit and overall intent of these laws. Because most managers are not directly involved in setting company policies and procedures, it is rare for them to need to consult with attorneys about how best to comply with existing statutes. If, however, you are asked to establish or enforce such organizational policies, it is a good idea to seek a legal review of these policies before they are adopted. A brief discussion of some of the legal issues that may be applicable to wellness follows.

The Americans with Disabilities Act (ADA)

The ADA requires employers to be careful not to discriminate against an employee on the basis of that individual's actual or perceived disability. Employers must offer reasonable accommodation to an employee with a disability. For example, fitness facilities must find ways to accommodate all employees. Similarly, wellness goals and rewards should be adjusted so that all can achieve success.

The ADA also prohibits employers from making medical inquiries or requiring medical examinations (unless they are job-related and consistent with business necessity). The Equal Employment Opportunity Commission has clarified this ADA rule. An employer may conduct voluntary medical examinations and activities that are part of a voluntary wellness and health screening program as long as there is no penalty for not participating. Any information acquired must be kept confidential.

The Employee Retirement Income Security Act (ERISA)

ERISA covers any program established to provide medical care to participants. While some wellness programs exclusively promote healthy lifestyles, many conduct individual health assessments and make specific recommendations to participants. These activities make a wellness program subject to ERISA, so they must comply with rules for claims procedures, summary plan descriptions and other ERISA requirements.

The Health Insurance Portability and Accountability Act (HIPAA)

HIPAA primarily governs the behavior of employers and service providers that offer health insurance. Nondiscrimination provisions prohibit companies from denying benefits on the basis of health factors and from charging higher premiums based on a health factor. However, a wellness program that offers incentives for certain behavior is likely to be in compliance with the law. You could, for example, offer incentives for physical activity as long as you accommodate people whose disability would make physical activity difficult. Such incentives also need to be less than 20 percent of the total cost of employee-only coverage.

National Labor Relations Act

Employers who have negotiated a collective bargaining agreement are required to bargain over wages, hours and other terms and conditions of employment. This generally means that the union should sign off on wellness program offerings, particularly if these programs have an impact on health insurance premiums.

State Laws That Protect Off-Duty Conduct

Some states have laws prohibiting employment discrimination as a result of lawful activity away from the employer's premises during nonworking hours. If your program will reward or penalize employees for activities outside work, you should determine whether state laws prohibit such activities.

General Principles to Keep in Mind to Avoid Legal Complications

A spirit of cooperation, nondiscrimination and kindness can do much to reduce the likelihood of legal complications. Where possible, adopt the following general operating principles.

- Do not collect or publicize individual and private information. Keep information anonymous and confidential. Base your efforts on group data and group goals that do not depend upon individual-level information.

- Use independent professional services to deliver individual assessments, incentives and counseling. This will help clear you of any concerns about employment discrimination.

- Find ways to make wellness programs accessible to all employees and accommodate the special needs of employees seeking to participate in wellness programs.

- Limit your use of incentives and penalties; these may become complicated by state and federal law. These types of initiatives should focus only on behavior and participation. Avoid linking them to health outcomes.

- Take employee concerns about the wellness program seriously. Listen and try to rectify problems that are posed, particularly if an employee is raising issues of fairness.

- Let employees know that the purpose of the wellness program is primarily to reduce barriers to healthy lifestyles and that the program is organized to support employees' efforts to achieve their own lifestyle goals. De-emphasize aspects of the wellness program that use guilt, fear or shame to push people toward specific wellness goals. Work with the existing lifestyle improvement interests of employees.

- Avoid heavy-handed tactics and any approach that seems unfair or burdensome. Remember that people's jobs are extremely important to their emotional and financial well-being. Any threat to employment is likely to invoke a negative reaction.

References

Note: References are offered in order of appearance in the *Wellness Leadership* text

A Call to Wellness Leadership

McGinnis JM, Foege WH. Actual causes of death in the United States. *Journal of the American Medical Association.* 1993;270:2207-2212.

Mokdad AH, Marks JS, Stroup DF, Gerberding JL. Actual causes of death in the United States, 2000. *Journal of the American Medical Association.* 2004;291:1238-1245.

McGinnis JM, Foege WH. The immediate vs the important. *Journal of the American Medical Association.* 2004;291:1263-1264.

Anderson RN, Smith BL. Deaths: leading causes for 2002. *National Vital Statistics Report.* 53(17). National Center for Health Statistics, March 7, 2005.

Allen J. 1984. Correlates of success in lifestyle change efforts. Paper presented at the 92nd annual meeting of the American Psychological Association, Toronto, Canada.

Allen J. 2001. Building supportive cultural environments. In *Health Promotion in the Workplace*, Michael P. O'Donnell, editor, Third Edition. 202-217. Delmar Publishers, Inc.

Aldana SG. 2005. *The Culprit & the Cure: Why Lifestyle Is the Culprit Behind America's Poor Health and How Transforming That Can Be the Cure.* Mapleton, UT: Maple Mountain Press.

Flegal KM, Carroll MD, Ogden CL. Prevalence and trends in obesity among US adults. *Journal of the American Medical Association.* 2002;288:1723-1727.

Centers for Disease Control and Prevention. Prevalence of physical activity, including lifestyle activities among adults: United States, 2000-2001. *MMWR.* 2003;52(32):764-769.

Sedula MK, Gillespie C, Kettel-Khan L, Farris R, Seymour J, Denny C. Trends in fruits and vegetables consumption among adults in the United States: Behavioral risk factor surveillance system, 1994-2000. *American Journal of Public Health.* 2004;94:1014-1018.

Pelletier KR. A review and analysis of the clinical and cost-effectiveness studies of comprehensive health promotion and disease management programs at the worksite: 1995-1998 update (IV). *American Journal of Health Promotion.* 1999;13:333-345.

Aldana SG. Financial impact of health promotion programs: A comprehensive review of the literature. *American Journal of Health Promotion.* 2001;15:296-320.

Goetzel RZ, Juday TR, Ozminkowski RJ. What's the ROI? A systematic review of the return-on-investment studies of corporate health and productivity management initiatives. *Worksite Health.* 1999;6(3):12-21.

Linnan L, Weiner B, Graham A, Emmons K. Manager beliefs regarding worksite health promotion: Findings from the Working Healthy Project 2, *American Journal of Health Promotion.* 2007;21(6):521-528.

Creating a Shared Wellness Vision

Dunn HL. High-level wellness for man and society. *American Journal of Public Health.* 1959;49(6):786-792.

Travis JW, Ryan RS. 2004. *Wellness Workbook: How to Achieve Enduring Health and Vitality.* Third Edition. Berkeley, CA: Celestial Arts.

Ardell DB. 1976. *High Level Wellness: An Alternative to Doctors, Drugs and Disease. Emmaus,* PA: Rodale.

Allen RF, Linde S. 1981. *Lifegain: The Exciting New Program That Will Change Your Health—and Your Life.* Burlington, VT: www.healthyculture.com.

Burton WN, Chen C, Conti DJ, Schultz AB, Edington DW. The association between health risk change and presenteeism change. *Journal of Occupational and Environmental Medicine.* 2006;48(3):252-263.

Pelletier KR. A review and analysis of the clinical and cost-effectiveness studies of comprehensive health promotion and disease management programs at the worksite: 1995-1998 update (IV). *American Journal of Health Promotion.* 1999;13:333-345.

Aldana SG. Financial impact of health promotion programs: A comprehensive review of the literature. *American Journal of Health Promotion.* 2001;15:296-320.

Goetzel RZ, Juday TR, Ozminkowski RJ. What's the ROI? A systematic review of the return-on-investment studies of corporate health and productivity management initiatives. *Worksite Health.* 1999;6(3):12-21.

Allen J, Hunnicutt D, Johnson, J. (1999). Fostering wellness leadership: A new model. *Special Report from the Wellness Councils of America.* Omaha, Nebraska

Serving as an Effective Role Model

Bandura A. 1977. *Social Learning Theory.* Englewood Cliffs, NJ: Prentice-Hall.

Allen J. 2008. *Healthy Habits, Helpful Friends: How to Effectively Support Wellness Lifestyle Goals.* Burlington, VT: www.healthyculture.com.

Allen J. 2002. The role of mentoring in health promotion. *The Art of Health Promotion.* 2002;6(4):1-12.

Aligning Cultural Touch Points

Allen J. 2008. *Healthy Habits, Helpful Friends: How to Effectively Support Wellness Lifestyle Goals.* Burlington, VT: www.healthyculture.com.

Allen RF, Kraft C. 1980. *Beat the System! A Way to Create More Human Environments.* New York, NY: McGraw-Hill.

Allen RF, Kraft C, Allen J, Certner B. 1987. *The Organizational Unconscious: How to Create the Corporate Culture You Want and Need.* Burlington, VT: www.healthyculture.com.

Monitoring and Celebrating Success

Goetzel RZ, Anderson DR, Whitmer RW, Ozminkowski RJ, Dunn RL, Wasserman J. The relationship between modifiable health risks and health care expenditures: An analysis of multi-employer HERO health risk cost database. *Journal of Occupational and Environmental Medicine.* 1998;40(10):843-854.

Allen J. 2001. Building supportive cultural environments. In *Health Promotion in the Workplace,* Michael P. O'Donnell, editor, Third Edition. 202-217. Albany, NY: Delmar Publishers, Inc.

Full Engagement

Allen J. 2001. Building supportive cultural environments. In *Health Promotion in the Workplace,* Michael P. O'Donnell, editor, Third Edition. 202-217. Albany, NY: Delmar Publishers, Inc.

Allen RF, Kraft C. 1980. *Beat the System! A Way to Create More Human Environments.* New York, NY: McGraw-Hill.

Allen RF, Kraft C, Allen J, Certner B. 1987. *The Organizational Unconscious: How to Create the Corporate Culture You Want and Need.* Burlington, VT: www.healthyculture.com.

Also by Judd Allen, Ph.D.

Bringing Wellness Home Bringing Wellness Home: How to Create a Household Subculture that Supports Wellness Lifestyle Goals is for anyone living with others. Very few lifestyle goals can be achieved without support at home. *Bringing Wellness Home* guides efforts to:

- Choose the household wellness norms you want and need.

- Create a shared vision for wellness at home.

- Align cultural influences such as traditions and rewards.

- Develop peer support skills that nurture positive and lasting lifestyle change.

- Foster a caring and fun household climate.

Healthy Habits, Helpful Friends: How to Effectively Support Wellness Lifestyle Goals empowers peers to assist with lifestyle change. In addition to learning how to lay a solid foundation for effective peer support, readers learn skills for: (1) setting wellness goals, (2) locating ideal role models, (3) eliminating barriers to change, (4) finding or creating supportive environments, (5) avoiding relapse, and (6) celebrating success. *Healthy Habits, Helpful Friends* serves as a text for Wellness Mentor Training.

Wellness Leadership, Bringing Wellness Home and *Healthy Habits, Helpful Friends* are available from the Human Resources Institute as a paperback and as an audiobook for $14.95. The books can be ordered at www.healthyculture.com. Call (802) 862-8855 to order the audiobook and for information about volume discounts.

Quick Book Order Form

For *Wellness Leadership, Bringing Wellness Home* and *Healthy Habits, Helpful Friends*

$14.95 each. Any two books for $24.95. Call for quantity pricing. US Shipping: $3.95 for first book. Fee shipping on additional US orders. $9 charge for the first two books shipped outside the US.

Please add 8% sales tax for books shipped to a Vermont address.

Quantity: ____ Wellness Leadership ____ Bringing Wellness Home

____ Healthy Habits, Helpful Friends

Name

Address

Billing address if other than shipping address

Telephone

Email

We gladly accept checks in U.S. funds payable to the Human Resources Institute, LLC

MasterCard or VISA Card Number _____

Expiration date _____

Fax orders: 802-862-6389

Telephone orders: 802-862-8855

Email orders: Info@healthyculture.com

Send postal orders to Healthyculture.com, 151 Dunder Road, Burlington, Vermont, 05401 USA

8422992R0

Made in the USA
Charleston, SC
08 June 2011